YOGA
FOR
ATHLETES

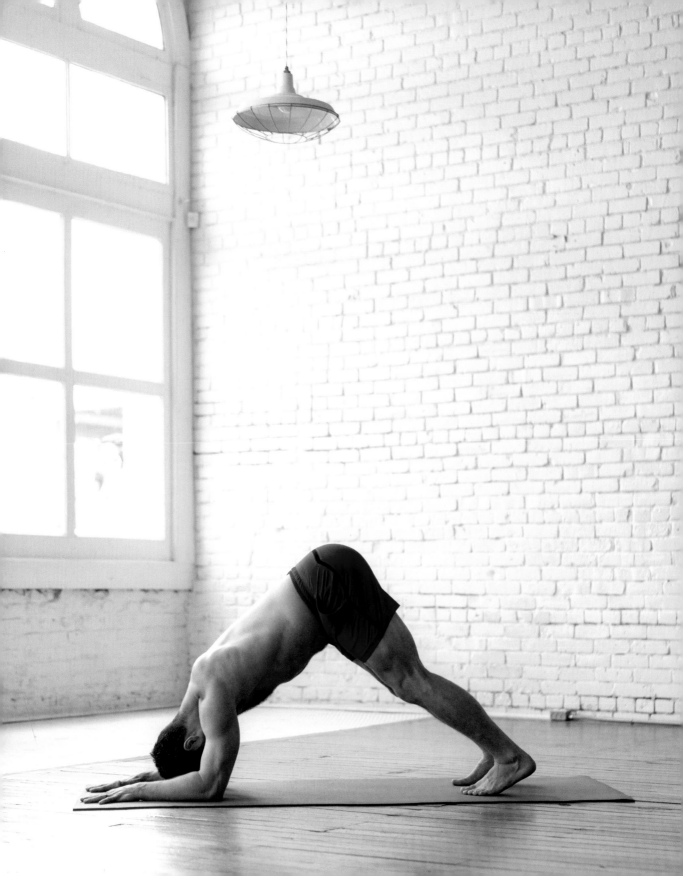

DEAN POHLMAN

YOGA

FOR

ATHLETES

10-MINUTE YOGA WORKOUTS TO MAKE YOU BETTER AT YOUR SPORT

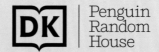

Publisher Mike Sanders
Senior Editor Alexandra Andrzejewski
Art & Design Director William Thomas
Senior Designer Jessica Lee
Photographer Dennis Burnett
Proofreader Lisa Starnes
Indexer Brad Herriman

First American Edition, 2021
Published in the United States by DK Publishing
6081 E. 82nd Street, Indianapolis, IN 46250

Copyright © 2021 by Man Flow Yoga LLC
DK, a Division of Penguin Random House LLC
21 22 23 24 25 10 9 8 7 6 5 4 3 2 1
001-323163-DEC2021

Library of Congress Catalog Number: 2021930990
ISBN 978-0-7440-3489-9

DK books are available at special discounts when purchased in bulk for
sales promotions, premiums, fund-raising, or educational use.
For details, contact: SpecialSales@dk.com

Printed and bound in Canada

Images (except for those credited on page 176) © Dorling Kindersley Limited

For the curious
www.dk.com

CONTENTS

FOREWORD

I'm not a small person. Don't get me wrong, I hang out with some really huge athletes, so I know what big really is. But, I'm still not small. Not small enough to sit for eight hours of lectures and presentations in a tiny plastic chair in a big conference hall. Like many of you, I'm that guy who usually stands in the back of the room or sits on the floor. My CEO/wife would tell you that I'm a little ADHD or that I hate organized fun, so being able to fidget or escape in the back of a packed lecture hall is really just who I am. (This aside will bear fruit; I promise.) But still, I'm playing the "big man" card.

A few years ago, I was attending a large digital marketing conference with our staff and true to my pattern, I found myself in an out-of-the-way corner of the vast conference room and popped down to listen (blissfully untrapped by one of those crappy venue bulk chairs). As I started to get my bearings and look around, I noticed a quite jacked-looking guy sitting in a not too socially awkward middle splits position next to me. Clearly I was in the right place.

You can guess who that person was in the back. That's right—Dean. For the next few days, it was clear that our interests in this conference were aligned. We kept meeting in the back of the room like two Cheerios in a big bowl of air-conditioned, carpeted, fluorescent-light milk hell. It helped that I already knew "famous Dean" from *Man Flow Yoga*, as I was already a fan. But is it too weird to say we found love in a hopeless place (thank you, Rhianna . . .)? You see, I already grokked Dean. I understood his model; the way he spoke and taught already worked for me.

Yoga is amazing. Has it also been co-opted a bit? Sure. Do I identify with most yoga communities? Not so much.

I don't want to trigger you here if you are a bad-ass yogi. But, yoga is simultaneously a brilliant movement system that is not messing around, and an excuse to never get under real load. Look, people have been trying to solve the problems of the common human condition for as long as there have been, well, humans. But yoga, like running, is sort of an incomplete "physical practice." Want to see how your standalone yoga practice is working for you? Here, carry this 100 pound sandbag up this hill. Yes, you have to pick it up off the ground . . .

If you speak pilates, Olympic weight lifting, kettlebells, Feldenkrais, or really any formal human movement system, then yoga makes perfect . . . crazy, intuitive sense. Yoga as a model to integrate breathing and foundational human movement shapes is at face value irrefutable. Think your "secret squirrel" strength and conditioning or fitness program is legit? Jump into a yoga program and test yourself. One, or zero. Yes, or no. You can stand on one leg or express hip extension and rotation, or you can't. Downward Dog is normative baseline hip flexion with the legs straight. And yes, if you have the dorsiflexion that every doctor on the planet agrees you should have when your leg is straight and your quads are flexed, your heels will be on the ground. Did you know Malasana is a fancy Sanskrit word for "squat." What do you mean you can't do yoga? Errrr, I mean squat.

So let me circle back to being a big guy that doesn't like organized fun. Oh, you mean a potential yoga class where *no* one looks like me? To me, this has been one of yoga's big stumbling blocks. My wife and I sometimes drop into our local "hot" yoga spot with some friends on the weekend. I use it as sort of a "truth" test. If my fitness and physical practices are legit, then dropping into a class

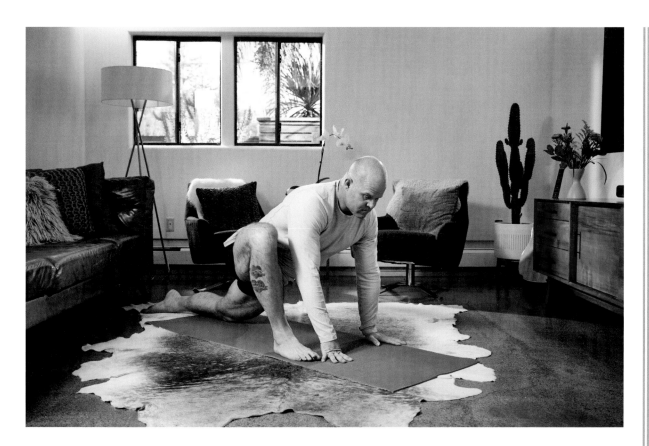

should be easy, right? After about the third or fourth time I went, the instructor grabbed me on the way out of the studio. "Hey, tell me what you do?" Me: "Well, among other things, I have a breath practice, I mobilize, and I spend time in the sauna." Her: "Oh, you are a yogi!" I loved that response. Most of the time I don't feel like I can commit to going to a yoga studio three to five times week and, still lift, bike, paddle, run, etc. The tenets of yoga—breath, positional competency, balance? Every day.

This is what makes Dean's work so great. To benefit from his coaching and programming, you definitely don't have to be a yogi. In fact, Dean would probably appreciate it if you were a little more well rounded and could dead lift two times your bodyweight. But, Dean has taken what is essential to our bodies, brains, and minds, and created a model based on the principles of a yogic practice—yoga as means to own positions and expose our tissues in places and ranges where we could use exposure and tolerance was always the game. Dean understands this

totally. You can drop this excellent book into whatever sport, practice, class, or activity you love, and it will make you better. I suspect that the majority of my professional career as a physiotherapist and performance coach to the world's best teams, organizations, and athletes would have been unnecessary if Dean's book was part of the plan.

Yoga is a kind of unified field theory of human movement. Let me say it again: people have been obsessed with solving the problems of the human condition for as long as there have been human beings. What we've all been missing is a way to work it into our busy lives. What we've been missing is a way to deploy the tactics of a full-throttled badass yoga practice into the sports and activities we love. What we've been missing is a teacher. So please, let me introduce to you my teacher, Dean Pohlman.

Dr. Kelly Starrett

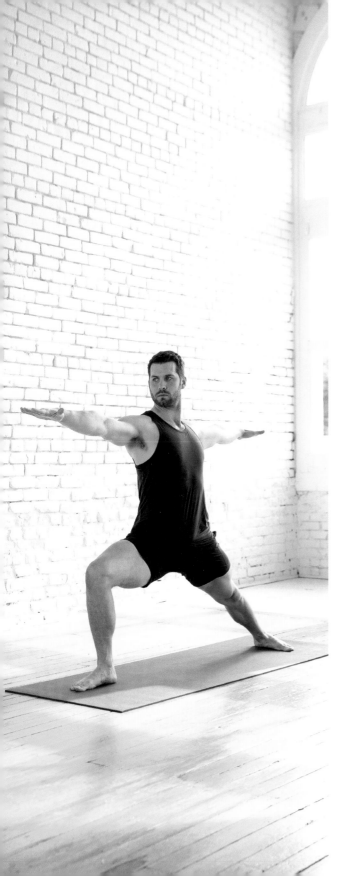

AN ATHLETE WHO DOES YOGA

I'm not a yogi posing as an athlete. I've been an athlete my entire life. Yoga came later on when I began to understand how it could help me be a better athlete—to be better at what I already did.

I don't want you to give up your other workouts and start doing five weekly 60-minute yoga sessions. I want to show you how just a few short yoga routines on a weekly basis can dramatically improve what you're already doing and teach you yoga in a way that makes sense. *Yoga for Athletes* is yoga on *your* terms.

Yoga found me when I wasn't looking for it. It had always intrigued me as something that could help me get stronger in new ways, but as a lifelong athlete and (at the time) a collegiate lacrosse player, I was already in excellent physical shape. I lifted weights regularly, conditioned on my own time, and was always first to the finish line in team sprints and agility drills. However, flexibility was something new to me. I didn't practice balancing skills. My idea of recovery was sitting on the couch and waiting for the soreness to go away.

As much as I was interested in the potential benefits yoga had to offer, I had no desire to go to a yoga studio. The only reason I ended up starting yoga was completely by accident—one day, while looking for the tailor, I stumbled into a yoga studio.

I was already on my way to work out afterward, so I thought I would give this a shot instead. The next 90 minutes were—and still are—the most challenging workout I've ever done. By the time we reached the halfway point, I was completely exhausted and looking around the room as if the cameras were going to come out at any moment and reveal I was being filmed for a prank TV show. But I wasn't being pranked. Those 90 minutes helped me understand just how weak I was in certain aspects of my fitness. I resolved to make yoga into a habit so I could continue to get stronger in new ways.

MEET THE CONTRIBUTORS

Get your yoga game in tip-top shape with these three athletes at the peak of their game.

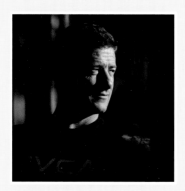

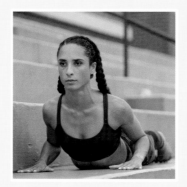

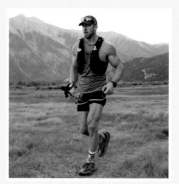

Brian Mackenzie is an elite athlete pushing the frontiers of physical fitness with innovative protocols for stress adaptation and breath work. Look for his expert contributions in the book to improve your own breathing patterns.
brianmackenzie.com

Francheska Martinez, at the top of her game in mobility and strength, helps athletes reach optimal functional movement. In addition to modeling yoga technique throughout the book, Francheska also chimes in with best practices so you, too, can become a strong, accomplished, mobile athlete.
francheskamartinez.com

Nick Bare, a hybrid elite athlete with a passion for pushing himself to peak fitness, knows what the body is capable of with proper training in the world of endurance and mobility. Nick will coach you through yoga for the endurance athlete so you can reach your full, staggering athletic potential.
nickbare.com

Over the next few months, I started branching out, attending different yoga studios, and trying different types of yoga classes. I loved the workouts and the postures, but there was one glaring aspect that just didn't jive with me; the workouts rarely focused on proper technique and how to do a little bit better each time.

What is the proper technique? What are the target areas? How is this posture benefiting me? These are the questions that ran through my head as I listened to yoga instructors who walked around the room discussing chakras, giving unsolicited life advice, and occasionally reminding me to breathe (this last part was very helpful and important). Most of the instruction I received was based on attempting to mirror what others did.

Eventually I started teaching yoga myself. As I developed my teaching style and interacted with my audience, I realized the questions I had as an early yoga practitioner were the same questions being asked by others. The more I taught, the more I realized I was essentially teaching the younger version of myself what I would have wanted when I had gotten started. And that is exactly what the goal of this book is—to teach you yoga, through the lens of an athlete, for you, an athlete.

Get stronger in new ways. Focus on breath work, recovery, balance, and mobility. **Get better at the sport you are already doing.** Choose from thirty 10-minute workouts specifically designed for your athletic needs. **Learn in a way that makes sense to your fitness goals.** Technique guides with detailed cues and helpful photographs teach you to make the most of every pose. Here you go—yoga *for* athletes, by an athlete. Really.

-Dean Pohlman

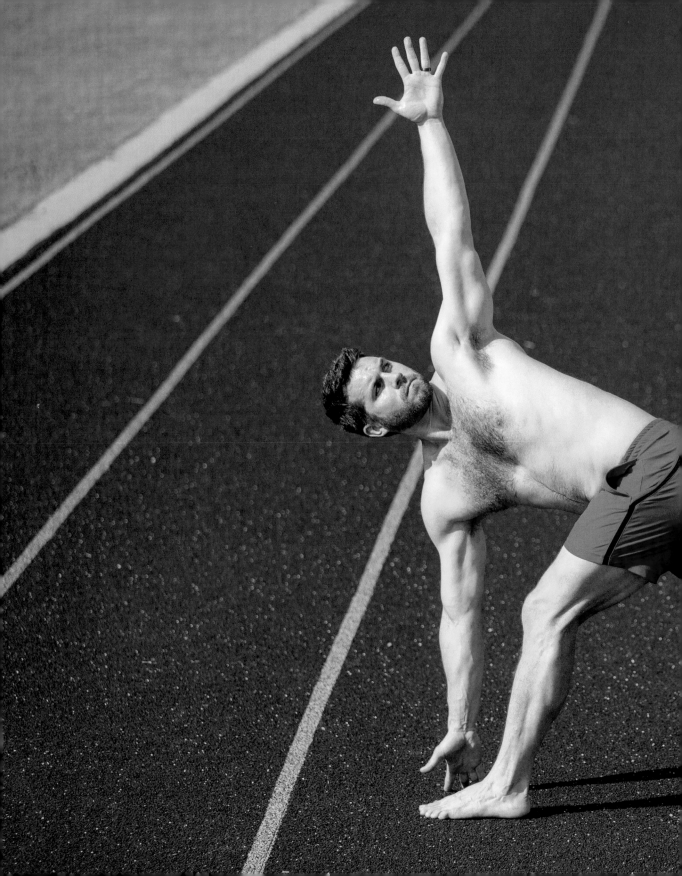

CHAPTER 1

FUNCTIONAL YOGA

PERFECT FOR ATHLETES

All those benefits you've heard about yoga are true. It can help tremendously with flexibility, joint health, longevity, and recovery. There is a reason why yoga is so commonly practiced by athletes, and that is because the benefits are noticeable—and often immediately. There are very few types of fitness that address such a wide range of benefits as does yoga when practiced effectively.

YOU SHOULD BE DOING YOGA

Increasing flexibility, decreasing recovery time, and preventing injury are some of the most common benefits as they relate to your athletic performance, but there are many other benefits you'll appreciate once you make yoga a consistent part of your workout routine.

Many of the benefits of yoga are cyclical and overlapping: they naturally build on one another, and the compounding nature of this growth is nothing short of dramatic. I haven't even included in my list all those aspects that support your general well-being, such as lowered blood pressure, heightened focus, improved immune support, and decreased anxiety and depression, but you can look forward to these as well with consistent practice.

The list of direct benefits goes on and on, and the list of indirect benefits is even longer. Either way you look at it, there's a whole bunch of reasons why practicing yoga should be a regular part of every athlete's weekly routine.

If you've heard anything about yoga, you're probably already familiar with its following benefits to your athletic performance:

BALANCE → Prevent injury; build strength; improve joint stability

FLEXIBILITY → Less strain on joints; faster recovery time; more fluid movements; decreased risk of injury

INJURY-PREVENTION → Dramatically lower risk of preventable soft-tissue injuries; skip fewer workouts; keep doing what you enjoy doing without pain

JOINT HEALTH → Less joint pain or discomfort during or after exercise; lowered risk of joint injuries; less wear and tear on the body over time

LONGEVITY → Enjoy your sport for as long as you possibly can, and at a higher performance level

RECOVERY → Get back to your workouts sooner with less soreness; reduced risk of injury from overtraining

And you might be surprised to learn about these other benefits to your performance:

BODY AWARENESS → Improved control over your body; better technique; improved muscle efficiency

BREATH WORK → Increased cardiovascular strength; ability to use your breath to control your body and control your stress response

EFFICIENCY → Lift more often; run faster; move better

MINDFULNESS → Make better decisions (both on and off the field, court, track, etc.)

MUSCLE ACTIVATION → Recruit more muscle fibers for much greater strength and power

SLEEP → Fall asleep more quickly to recover more quickly for your next workout and to get stronger more quickly

STRENGTH → Lift more weight; perform more reps

STRESS → Relax better when you're not working out; have greater awareness of your emotions; fall asleep easily; and even improve your hormone levels to better support your physical well-being so you feel your best for every workout

WHICH ATHLETES DOES THIS BOOK HELP?

Whatever you want to call yourself—weekend warrior, fitness enthusiast, workout junkie, member of the team, sports-person—you are an athlete (whether you think of yourself as one or not). Whether you're playing for fun or for medals, the common denominator is that you like a good sweat and you want to get better. Rather than delving into all of the specific types of sports out there, this book hones in on the two overarching areas of fitness—resistance training and endurance training. All athletes fall into one of these categories, and each earns a devoted chapter and suggested yoga workouts. Inevitably, there is overlap between the two, or you may be fully involved in both resistance and endurance training. You are encouraged to read the content from both sections . . . just use whatever seems most helpful for your goals.

Resistance Training (p. 24–35): anybody who lifts weights, does bodyweight exercises, goes to the gym, participates in CrossFit, etc. Content for this type of athlete focuses on how yoga can best complement any form of strength training, filling the gaps by addressing common weaknesses, providing much-needed recovery routines, and helping to avoid common injuries. Whether better lifting is your end goal, or if you're using it as conditioning to get better at a sport, yoga will help you.

Endurance Training (pages 36–47): runners, cyclists, triathletes, swimmers, rowers, etc. The content here helps endurance athletes complement their existing training routines. Address common issues like overtraining, correct imbalances caused by repetitive movements, and otherwise learn how to improve your performance and decrease your risk of injury.

There really is no workout or pose in this book that won't help you, regardless of your training of choice, but the individual workouts are meant to address the specific needs of their target athlete. I've taken special care to make sure that the workouts and content in this book are as relevant as possible without including content that, while generally helpful, is not specifically helpful for you.

Frequency of Your Practice

In order to reap the benefits of yoga, you must practice yoga consistently. My recommendation is to do at least four to six yoga workouts per week, or close to an hour of work. Considering you can easily insert yoga workouts into the beginning, middle, or end of your existing workouts (not to mention as a standalone routine), this is much easier than it seems—plus, the workouts in the book only take about 10 minutes. The return on investment is well worth it.

Prehabilitation, Not Rehabilitation

This is not meant to be a book on rehabilitation. There is a difference between exercises to help prevent knee injury, and exercises to recover from knee injury. Although many of these poses can help with rehabilitation once injury has been experienced, every case is unique. If you are already injured, consult a medical professional such as a physical therapist.

Addressing Your Apprehensions

Yoga does not have to be a lifestyle change or require you turn yourself into a pretzel. As a guy whose career is dedicated to helping other guys who wouldn't normally get started with yoga to get started with yoga, I fully understand the skepticism and fears. Maybe you're not interested in the spiritual stuff. You don't think you'll sweat enough. Maybe it's intimidating because you're not flexible and feel completely behind.

These apprehensions are completely legitimate. I've seen plenty of "beginner's" yoga classes that would only be helpful for a very flexible, advanced practitioner. I've seen yoga classes that are too easy and feel like an inefficient use of time. But just like fitness in general, there are a *lot* of ways to practice yoga. I want to show you yoga in a way that directly benefits you, an athlete, that makes you better at what you're already doing. This is truly yoga for athletes—nothing extra. In order to make yoga as athlete-centered as possible, read on to learn how you can practice yoga in a way that takes your fitness up a notch.

THE BIG TWO

Many athletes skip out on yoga because they assume it's just stretching, but to equate yoga to stretching classes is like simplifying endurance training to running around in circles on a track. There's a reason why athletes are turning to yoga more and more. The specific poses and the movement approach of yoga combine to form benefits that earn you a real bang for your buck—*if* you do it the right way with a focus on technique. What really makes yoga unique? The special sauce boils down to these two ingredients: breathing and mind-body awareness.

BREATHING

Does your breathing need work? Unless you practice breathing consciously, with deliberation, I'm here to say it does. At the heart of mindful movement is the recognition that breathing controls your body. It is in integrating mindful movement with the inhales and exhales of your breath that you pull together the magic of yoga. If you're out of breath, you lose control. If your inhales and exhales are slow, steady, and synced with your movement, you can maintain control. Of course, if you're exerting yourself 100 percent, you're going to reach a point where you can no longer maintain control of your breathing, but practicing your breathing allows you to push the limits of what that maximum range is.

The relationship between your body and your breathing controls your body's fight-or-flight response. It facilitates a dialogue between your body and your brain—when your body says "no, we can't do this," your mindful exhalation says "relax, yes we can." This is a very important concept when it comes to increasing flexibility. Once you fully realize—both intellectually and practically—your ability to release muscle tension from the body through your breath, your flexibility and recovery work skyrocket in effectiveness. You'll be able to release muscle stress in recovery workouts more effectively and get back to your workouts with less soreness. You can use your breathing to switch off the fight-or-flight response of your sympathetic nervous system and activate the rest-and-digest response of your parasympathetic nervous system. You'll also be able to use your breathing to work deeper into postures and to increase your overall flexibility so you can, in turn, increase your overall physical fitness.

Generally speaking, you will inhale to lengthen and expand your body and exhale to go deeper and relax further into the pose. In yoga, we use diaphragmatic breathing, or "belly breathing." Brian Mackenzie walks you through how to do that on page 16. Diaphragmatic breathing helps you fully use your diaphragm to make breathing effective and efficient. This helps you maintain the integrity of your posture, ensuring your hips, core, and shoulders remain in alignment. That means that just improving your breathing can improve your technique during your lifts, runs, etc., for less strain on your joints and better muscle engagement. The best way to get better at proper breathing during movement is to simply practice. The more you practice breathing in your yoga workouts, the more easily it will carry over into your other workouts. If you practice enough, one day you'll realize that you now do it subconsciously. Ask yourself again—is breathing really that important? Yeah, it is.

MIND-BODY AWARENESS

The basic idea behind mind-body awareness is motor control—being able to control the different parts of your body, knowing how to engage specific muscle groups, and being able to move mindfully. Mind-body awareness is typically absent in faster, athletic movements, but yoga gives you a great opportunity to practice it. Why should you care? Because mind-body awareness allows your muscles to work as efficiently as possible. It makes you stronger by allowing you to recruit more muscle fibers into your movements and get every bit of strength and power you can out of your muscles—especially when it counts! On top of that, practicing mind-body awareness also improves technique—in all of your movement! You'll have the presence of mind to check in while training and make sure that you're moving mindfully and efficiently, and avoiding improper movements that can lead to injury.

PUTTING IT ALL TOGETHER

You might be thinking "that's a whole lot to keep in mind." You're right—it can be challenging to remember to focus on breathing and proper technique all at once. That's one of the reasons why yoga is so effective at improving focus. It gives you the opportunity to laser focus your attention on these subtle aspects and completely block out the other random distractions that disrupt your thinking.

Here is a sample of what your inner dialogue might sound like. The pose we'll use is a relatively basic one, Chair (p. 114), but you'll notice the fine-tuning of many details involved as you practice it.

BREATHING

"Use the inhale to get taller and lengthen my body."

"Use the exhale to bend deeper."

"Use the inhale to re-establish length after the exhale."

"Use the exhale to squeeze the abs and go deeper."

MIND-BODY AWARENESS

"I need to be sure to engage my abs to protect my back."

"Press down firmly into both feet so my body weight is evenly distributed in both legs."

"Make sure my butt is out and back, glutes are engaged, and lower back isn't rounding."

"Don't get lazy with the arms. Keep my arms squeezing up and back so my shoulders are opening up and upper back muscles are engaged."

All of these thoughts might go through your head as you practice yoga. It's what makes it so effective. If that seems overwhelming at first, know that it takes repetition. You won't be able to do all of this at once, but you can slowly implement one aspect at a time until one day you're going through the checklist in your head, making sure you're doing all of the things you can be doing to make sure you're getting the most effective use of your time.

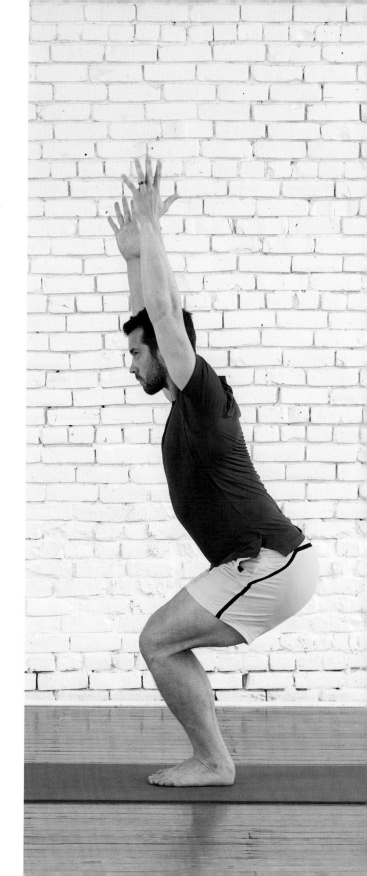

BREATH WORK
WITH GUEST COACH BRIAN MACKENZIE

Yoga is the oldest movement practice we know of. It's rooted in many fundamentals that apply to today's exercise science and physiological principles. At the foundation of these principles is a term in Sanskrit: *pranayama.* Broken down, the word means *to control the breath.* That means energy control—all energy begins and ends from breath. Breath is yoga's foundation, and it isn't just woo-woo; this understanding comes from well-established scientific principles.

IMPORTANCE OF BREATHING

Physiologically speaking, breathing is the most potent and easily accessible way to control your nervous system, namely your autonomic nervous system (ANS). In conjunction with the ANS, your breathing directly impacts aerobic and anaerobic cellular respiration. Aerobic cellular respiration is the most efficient means we understand for transferring energy, and breath control teaches us exactly how to make this more efficient.

Psychologically, when we have more control over our nervous system due to breath control, we automatically bring on more parasympathetic activity. This has largely been known as the "rest, digest, and reproduce" side of our ANS, but much more than that, it provides an ability to clearly feel and think through many of the things going on in our restless minds. It is an access point to creativity, calmness, and better sleep quality.

Our breathing controls how we "organize" ourselves mechanically from the diaphragm, which circumnavigates the bottom of our rib cage and spine. If the diaphragm struggles to work well, we are "disorganized" and compensate with poor movement. This is the beauty and idea of yoga: move and work with your breath, never moving faster than the energy we can control. Breath provides us with the first stages of what a practice is, the journey of oneself, through oneself, to find oneself.

APPLYING BREATH WORK

You can use your breathing as a barometer to determine the appropriate level of depth you should strive for in each yoga posture.

- You should be able to draw a full breathing cycle from inhale to exhale as much as possible in the pose, even if it's a challenging posture. Note that this will be limited in some poses, and that is perfectly fine.

- Take time at the top of an inhale to pause before exhaling, and notice what this does for your body awareness and the pose.

- Do your best to complete the full breath cycle in and out of the nose (nasal breathing). When the workout is significantly challenging, you may have to use your mouth to breathe.

- Pay particular attention to the positioning of your ribcage. You should be able to feel your ribs expanding in all directions horizontally as you inhale.

- If you do not feel the breath in a particular area (say, the upper back) by maintaining the above cues, concentrate drawing a breath into and out of that area.

Here is how to practice.

1. Come into a comfortable seated or standing position with your spine neutral.

2. Tuck your chin, and pull the top of your head tall.

3. Anchor your rib cage flat by slightly contracting your abdominal wall.

4. Start breathing slowly in and out.

5. Pay attention to your thoracic positioning:

   - Externally rotate your palms to face forward, and organize your shoulders.

   - Feel the movement in your rib cage in all horizontal

directions when breathing (i.e. feel your rib cage expanding in all directions as you breathe in).

- Avoid overly arching or puffing out your chest. Otherwise, you'll notice breathing in the front of your chest is restricted.

- Avoid internal rotation of your shoulders. Otherwise, you limit your thoracic mobility, and breathing in the back of your ribs will be restricted.

6. Pay attention to your pelvic floor and core engagement:

- As you inhale, concentrate on expanding your diaphragm in all directions to fill your lower pelvic floor with air, all the way from the base of your trunk to the tops of your ribs. Your pelvic floor should be relaxed, and transverse abdominals lightly engaged. You should feel your inner thighs and pelvic floor lightly resist the diaphragm expansion in the inhale.

- As you exhale, lightly squeeze your transverse abdominals. This facilitates engagement of the pelvic floor and inner thigh muscles, bringing your hips toward one another. Your pelvic floor should be engaged as if you were stopping yourself from going to the bathroom.

POSTURES TO PRACTICE DIAPHRAGMATIC BREATHING

Use the following postures in the prescribed order to put diaphragmatic breathing into action.

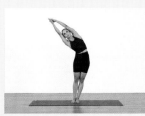

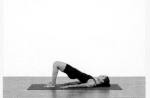

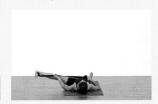

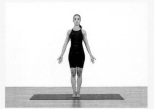

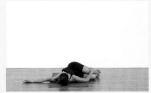

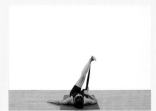

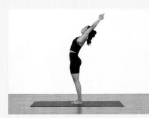

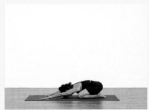

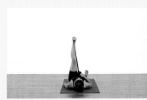

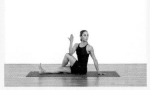

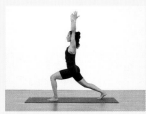

Mountain (p. 136)
10 breaths

Bridge (p. 110)
5 breaths

Child's Pose (p. 116)
5 breaths

High Lunge (p. 130)
5 breaths per side

Seated Twist (p. 148)
3 breaths per side

Reclined Twist (p. 144)
3 breaths per side

Hamstring Strap Stretch (p. 142)
5 breaths per side

Adductor Strap Stretch (p. 142)
5 breaths per side

Abductor Strap Stretch (p. 142)
5 breaths per side

Standing Sidebend (p. 158)
3 breaths per side

Standing Backbend (p. 154)
5 breaths

HOW TO IMPLEMENT ATHLETE-CENTERED YOGA

There are many different ways to practice yoga, and that means there are multiple ways to integrate it into your existing training schedule. Here is how you can use the content in this book to advance your athleticism.

USING THIS BOOK

1. Read through "Chapter 1: Functional Yoga." Familiarize yourself with athlete-centered yoga. This is helpful for a few reasons. First, learning about the benefits motivates you to actually use these workouts and postures. Second, you'll need to practice yoga in a specific way to reap noticeable results instead of just mirroring the postures and hoping for the best.

2. Explore your specific weaknesses, and diagnose areas of growth with the "Posture Assessment Guide" (pp. 21–23). The assessment walks you through five yoga postures to help you measure strength and mobility in the major muscle groups and joints of your body—spine, shoulders, hips, and ankles. Almost all athletes will find areas of opportunity from this test, so you're sure to find something you can improve.

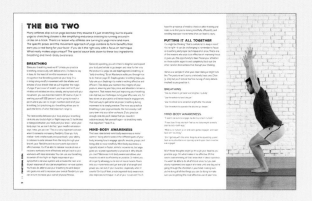

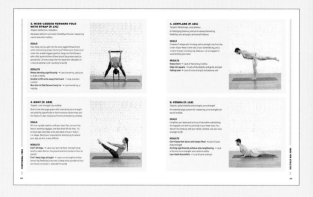

WHEN TO DO THE WORKOUTS

Some of the workouts in the book are multi-purposed, meaning you can use them as standalone workouts or as recovery workouts, while others have more specific uses. For the purposes of this book, you're instructed to apply the yoga workouts in three ways.

Warm-Ups: A series of strength and mobility postures to help improve muscle activation, work into your functional range of motion, and prepare your body for exercise. You can use these 10-minute routines immediately before your normal workouts to improve your performance, reduce strain on your joints, and move more fluidly.

Cooldowns and Recovery: Restorative stretches to help your body wind down, transition from the sympathetic nervous system to the parasympathetic nervous system, and jump-start the recovery process. You should do these workouts immediately following your workout when your muscles are still warm.

Standalone Workouts: Workouts you can do outside of your other fitness workouts (without being used

3. Jump to "Yoga for Resistance Training" (pp. 24–35) or "Yoga for Endurance Training" (pp. 36–47), depending on your fitness discipline of choice. Scan the chapter for topics that address your known weaknesses. Most athletes know they need to "work on their hip mobility" or "do more recovery workouts," so if you already know what you need to work on, find it, read up on it, and then check out the routine or poses that will best address that particular issue.

4. Follow the prescriptive workouts from chapters 2 or 3. These workouts are composed of the 34 yoga poses at the end of the book. In the routine, you'll find a thumbnail of each pose included, as shown below. For a more complete walk-through of each pose—including specific tips for breathing properly and building strength in the pose—flip to the pose section (organized in alphabetical order, pp. 104–171).

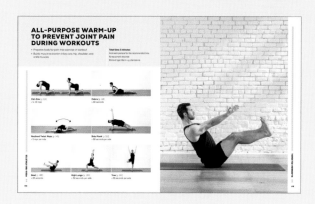

immediately before or after your other workouts) as a way to build strength and endurance, increase mobility and flexibility, and improve your balance. There are a few longer workouts in the book that are perfect for this, but the majority of these routines are about 10 minutes long. (And what athlete doesn't have time for a 10-minute workout?)

HOW TO DO THE POSES

Some yoga poses are great as a warm-up, while other poses are better suited toward a post-workout stretch …

some can do both, depending on how you do it! This book includes plenty of information to make sure you correctly pair the postures with what your body physically needs at the time. Postures can be practiced with different goals. It just depends on how you execute that pose; you could choose a variation or modification, or you can adjust the intensity or depth of the posture. (Once you try it for yourself, you'll see what I mean!) The same is generally true for other types of exercise. A run can be restorative if it's a gentle jog with shorter distance, but it can be extremely intense if you're pushing your limit and moving faster. Weight training with lower weights is a great way to actively recover, but doing the exact same exercises with higher weights can tax your body to its max.

For example, Child's Pose (p. 116) is very restorative if it's done at the end of a workout. It stretches your shoulders, helps you return your breathing to normal, and even puts your body into a position that helps activate the parasympathetic nervous system. On the other hand, you can perform child's pose more actively if you mobilize your shoulders and actively open your chest—this would be great prior to a workout that requires upright posture and fully engaged scapular stabilizers.

Here are some general guidelines on how to practice yoga for each situation.

Warm-Up: focus on active mobility and strength.

You want to concentrate on maintaining strength throughout the entire duration of the pose. As you do this, you should also work on going deeper into the pose, but not so much that you feel your muscles turn off and you only feel stretching. Avoid passive stretching and flexibility work during your warm-up, as this decreases performance. That means you'll also want to avoid supported or restorative versions of postures in which you rely on a wall, block, or other external support to help hold up your bodyweight.

You may (or may not) be surprised to learn that not all yoga is appropriate as a warm-up. Static stretching has actually been proven to decrease overall performance, so there are certain yoga postures you'll definitely want to avoid before an intense workout. (Although, if you are deciding between decreased performance and increased risk of injury due to muscle tightness and lack of mobility, I would recommend you choose the former.)

On the other hand, many postures found in yoga are great for warm-up because they help to activate your muscles, turning on your core, your hips, your back, and other areas that need to be engaged for proper exercise. Yoga is full of isometric positions, which is not only a great way to improve body awareness, but also to pump blood into the muscles and prepare them for exercise.

Cooldown and Recovery: focus on passive flexibility and stretching.

After your workout or for the purpose of recovery, you want to help the muscles to relax and release tension. This is where pose variations using blocks or supported against a wall come in handy because they facilitate a better release of tension.

During these more restorative routines, you'll want to minimize emphasis on strength and active mobility. After you've done a workout, your body is tired and you've probably already put it through the necessary amount of stress to help yourself grow stronger. Much more helpful during this time is to focus on your recovery, and you do that mainly through passive stretching.

Standalone Workouts: depending on the goals of the workout, you'll want to focus on different things.

However, here's the typical progression of a standalone yoga workout:

- Warm-Up: This can either be in the form of easier flexibility work to help you ease into the workout, or isometric-strengthening postures to help improve muscle activation and maximize your performance during the workout.

- Workout: This is where you should feel comfortable pushing yourself, both in the form of working deeper into the postures, as well as holding the postures to the point of failure (if you choose to do so).

- Cooldown (Optional): This is not included in every yoga routine, but if you do have restorative postures at the end of the routine, this is the time to focus on passive flexibility and restoration. Here, you'll want to slow down your breathing, relax your body, and do your best to release muscle tension.

Overall, there is really no time of day when a little bit of yoga here and there wouldn't be helpful, but it certainly helps to make sure that you are choosing the postures and routines that most complement your physical activity goals at that specific time.

POSTURE ASSESSMENT GUIDE

Use this guide to assess your current mobility levels, identify areas of opportunity, and help to identify potential weaknesses that could lead to issues down the road if left unaddressed. Note: Your mobility in your 20s is drastically different from your mobility in your 50s and beyond. Understanding mobility levels is helpful, but it's not the *only* way to measure your yoga fitness.

WHAT TO DO

These five postures help you measure your mobility, strength, and flexibility levels. Make sure you're using proper technique. Refer to the indicated pages for a more in-depth walk-through of proper posture technique. Do each pose in front of a mirror, or better yet, take a video of yourself and watch it later on. Ideally you will hold the pose with control for 5 to 10 seconds while maintaining good control of your breathing (breathing in and out of your nose without huffing and puffing). It's okay if your muscles are shaking. Qualitatively asses your posture with the results section to learn if you should focus on a particular weakness in the following chapters.

1. HORSE (P. 132)

Targets: hips, glutes, adductors

This is a great overall assessment of functional hip mobility. It measures the ability of your adductors to stretch while maintaining strength through your lower body.

GOALS

How low can you get into the horse squat while maintaining proper technique? Back should be mostly flat (a little bit of an arch is fine). Knees should track over your middle toes (not cave inward). Arches of feet should be pronounced (no pronation).

RESULTS

Feet turning in → Less adductor mobility
Knees caving in → Less adductor mobility
Back arched → Less adductor mobility, lack of glute engagement

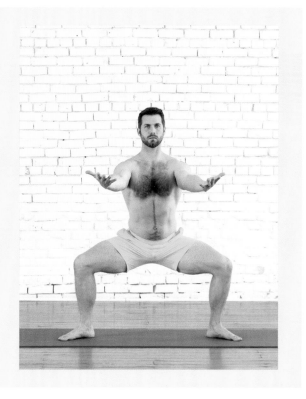

2. WIDE-LEGGED FORWARD FOLD: WITH STRAP (P. 171)

Targets: adductors, shoulders

Assesses adductor and ankle flexibility while also measuring overall shoulder mobility.

GOALS

How deep can you get into the wide-legged forward fold while maintaining proper technique? Widen your stance and come into a wide-legged position. Hinge and fold forward with a flat spine. Arches of feet should be pronounced (no pronation). Lift arms away from the back with shoulders in a neutral position (not rounding forward).

RESULTS

Knees bending significantly → Less hamstring, adductor, or ankle mobility
Unable to lift arms away from back → Less shoulder mobility
Not able to fold forward very far → Less hamstring or mobility

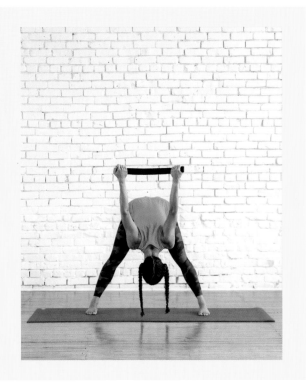

3. BOAT (P. 108)

Targets: core strength, hip mobility

Boat is the best yoga posture for evaluating core strength and stability, specifically in the transverse abdominals and hip flexors. It also measures functional hamstring mobility.

GOALS

Sit in an upright position with your back flat, core and hip flexors actively engaged, and feet lifted off the floor. Try to keep legs extended, arms extended, and your body in a V-shape. Bend your knees before attempting to extend your legs, as this is very difficult.

RESULTS

Can't lift legs → Less core and hip flexor strength (may need to place feet on the ground and rest hands on the floor to assist)
Can't keep legs straight → Less core strength and less hamstring flexibility (may need to keep shins parallel to floor and hands on knees or extended forward)

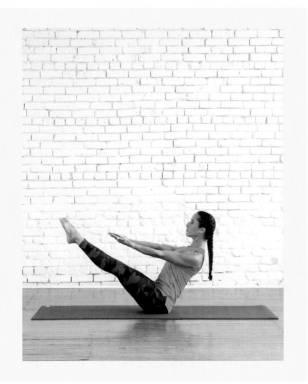

4. AIRPLANE (P. 104)

Targets: hamstrings, core, balance

A challenging balance posture to assess hamstring flexibility, core strength, and overall balance.

GOALS

Create a T-shape with your body, with a straight line from the crown of your head to the toes of your extended leg, and a mostly straight standing leg. Keep your core engaged to avoid arching your back.

RESULTS

Knees bent → Lack of hamstring mobility
Hips not square → Lack of hip stability and glute strength
Falling over → Lack of core strength and balance skill

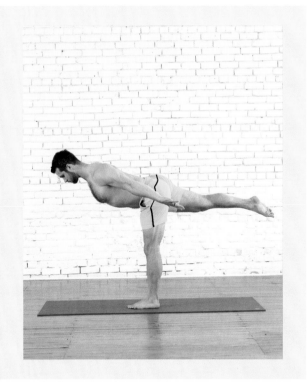

5. COBRA (P. 118)

Targets: spinal mobility and strength, core strength

An essential yoga posture for measuring core strength and spinal mobility.

GOALS

Lengthen your spine and arch your back while maintaining an engaged core with no pinching in your lower back. You should not press up with your hands. Instead, use your core strength to lift.

RESULTS

Can't keep feet down and knees lifted → Lack of lower body strength
Arching significantly without also lengthening → Lack of hip and core strength; poor spinal mobility
Lower back discomfort → Lack of core strength

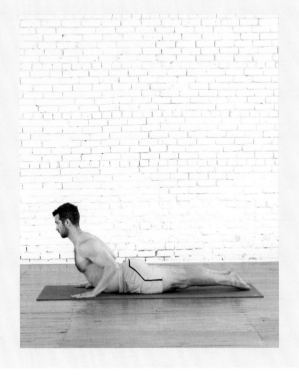

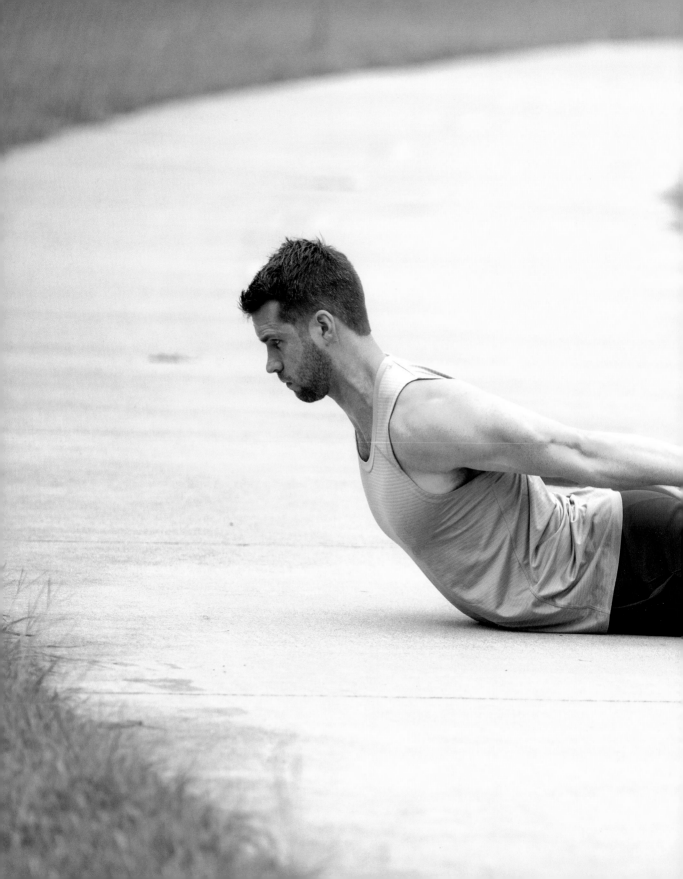

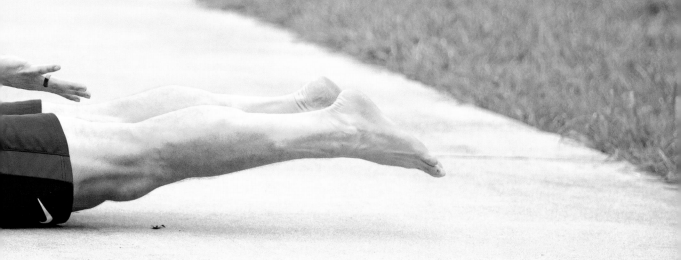

CHAPTER 2 »
YOGA FOR RESISTANCE TRAINING

THE RESISTANCE ATHLETE

Most strength trainers argue weight lifting is the most effective method for building strength and increasing overall muscle mass—and they're absolutely right. However, weight lifting itself does not address every aspect of fitness required for improving your overall physical performance—even if your goal is just to get better at weight lifting. Regularly doing yoga, both as a way to strengthen weaknesses and as recovery training to lock in your gains, can help you take your performance to the next level, lift more weight, and feel better while doing it.

USING THIS CHAPTER

To help you understand where your weaknesses lie, you will explore three categories of your fitness: common weaknesses, typical training gaps, and common pain points. Alongside an overview of these items, each specific topic covered will direct you to routines or specific postures that will help you address your goals. For example, as we discuss common shoulder injuries, that section also includes the postures and routines recommended to help prevent shoulder injury. Choose from the recommended workouts or poses to build your yoga practice. Aim to get in about six workouts per week. (Using the routines in this book, that adds up to just 60 minutes!)

CONSISTENCY AND RESULTS

If you can do 60 minutes of yoga per week, you should notice results within just four weeks—and most likely, even sooner. Your lifts will feel better, you'll have more awareness in your body, and you won't feel as sore the day after lifting. You need to keep it up to continue to notice the results! If you stop doing yoga, those noticeable improvements will start to go away within weeks.

HOW YOGA CAN HELP WITH RESISTANCE TRAINING

Your training probably has predictable gaps and common pain points. Here's an overview of what you have to look forward to with a targeted and consistent yoga practice.

» Decrease risk of preventable injuries, aches, and pains:

- Avoid injuries due to lack of mobility and flexibility
- Avoid injuries due to muscular imbalances and poor muscle activation

» Increase strength in commonly weak areas:

- Address smaller, less commonly worked muscles to build functional strength
- Correct muscular imbalances to reduce strain on joints
- Build isometric strength to build more overall strength
- Practice balance to build strength and stability in new ways

» Increase mobility and flexibility:

- Increase overall strength by improving functional range of motion
- Decrease risk of injury through increased flexibility and mobility
- Speed up recovery with increased flexibility

» Improve breathing:

- Improve overall athletic performance and strength with more efficient breathing
- Improve posture through proper breathing technique, which also lowers risk of injury
- Increase body awareness and mindfulness with intentional breathing

RESISTANCE TRAINING
WITH GUEST COACH FRANCHESKA MARTINEZ

Taking the time to learn how to balance both my strength and mobility training has been one of the best decisions of my athletic journey.

When I was in my late teens and early 20s, I was a bit of an extremist—I had phases when I would only do aerobics or mobility training and phases when I would focus primarily on strength, with little time spent in both worlds. You can bet that I had minor injuries and nagging pains.

Just like we know that cooling down is important but we skip it at the end of our work out, I knew I needed both strength and mobility in my training. It wasn't until I had a nagging shoulder injury that lasted well over a year that I realized I needed to make a drastic change. The nagging shoulder started when my training was imbalanced. I was spending too much time focusing on strength gains, and not properly recovering or spending time doing mobility exercises and stretching. Then I went to the other extreme where I stopped lifting weights completely for a few months. Once I took a break from strength training, I realized how crucial it was for maintaining my overall functional strength and particularly helping keep my core and joints strong, especially because I had some preexisting injuries and spine issues that seemed to worsen when I completely stopped weight lifting. That's when I started to become more methodical about my programming and become more conscientious about balancing both ends of the spectrum, making sure that I was strong and athletic as well as soft and malleable.

What made the biggest difference was filling in movement gaps and deficiencies in my training: smarter movement prep, more isometric body-weight work, and lots of spinal twists. Every body is different, but I am more than certain that every person can benefit from adding variety to their movement repertoire. Since the union of my mobility and strength training, I have never felt better. My training is focused on both performance and longevity, making sure that I'm always prioritizing joint and tissue health, as well as maintaining my range of motion and strength.

What's most rewarding about training in both worlds is seeing how it translates to other parts of my life, whether it be hiking, daily life, learning how to surf, or trying new physical activities. It always keeps my body primed, adaptable, and ready to take on any new challenges. Having a balanced practice has made it so that I can avoid injuries and recover faster, while still focusing on performing to my highest capacity.

Incorporating both strength and yoga into a training regimen is like having both yin and yang, softness and strength, to actualize our potential and abilities. A well-balanced athlete is someone who embodies and practices both strength and malleability—supplementing with yoga is good for your long-term health.

I recommend you start each yoga session like this:

1. **Imagine that you're about to perform a ballet on a stage.** Take a deep belly breath and visualize a string pulling you upward from the crown of your head.

2. **Remember that posture and mood are related!** So stand up with a broad chest, and think of a time that you felt most proud or happy.

3. **Find your tall neutral stance—Mountain (p. 136)— and breath.** Use this mental sequence:

   » Tuck your hips under, and find a neutral position.

   » Take in a deep belly breath, and exhale deeply.

   » Imagine a string pulling from the top of your head.

   » Roll your shoulders down and back.

   » Take in another deep belly breath, and exhale deeply.

   » Pull your neck back in line with spine. Relax your jaw.

   » Lastly, press your tongue against the roof of your mouth, and repeat a deep breath cycle.

WEAKNESSES

The following are some scenarios of weakness you might face: a lack of flexibility and mobility leads to improper technique, which places unnecessary strain on joints, causing imbalances that can lead to injury; a lack of muscle activation training holds back performance; not enough recovery work delays strength gains; and not enough attention to breathing hinders overall strength and performance. If you're a weight lifter who wants to optimize your overall performance, let's look at these common weaknesses—or as I like to think of them, the low-hanging fruits to improving our overall physical fitness.

LACK OF FLEXIBILITY & MOBILITY

Proper weight lifting necessitates a significant level of mobility. The issue for most weight-lifting athletes is they don't have this mobility to begin with, and they practice weight-lifting exercises without going through the full range of motion. The lack of mobility leads to imbalances, pain, and injury. Flexibility (the precursor to mobility) is the ability of your muscles to stretch into an extended range of motion. On the other hand, mobility is building strength within that extended range of motion. While flexibility is important for speeding up recovery and helping with overall injury prevention, weight lifters notice more performance benefits with mobility because this is what allows them to squat deeper with more weight, to feel stronger at the bottom of their dead lifts, and, in general, to lift without poor movement compensations that can cause excessive strain on the joints.

The table shows areas of inflexibility or immobility and their corresponding symptoms. **If you have any of the issues below, consider the recommended routines:**

INFLEXIBILITY » SYMPTOM	BUILD YOUR PRACTICE WITH THESE WORKOUTS
Hip inflexibility » Knee or back issues	Hip Strength & Mobility (p. 58) · Overall Hip Flexibility (p. 76) · Adductor & Hamstring Flexibility (p. 77) · Glute, Hip Flexor & Quadricep Flexibility (p. 78) · Knee Soreness Relief (p. 95) · Total Spine Relief (p. 99)
Limited range of motion in dead lifts » Lower-back pain or potential spinal injury	Resistance Athlete's Strength, Mobility, Flexibility & Balance (p. 68) · Full-Body Strength, Mobility & Injury Prevention (p. 72) · Overall Hip Flexibility (p. 76) · Adductor & Hamstring Flexibility (p. 77) · Compound Strength Movement Warm-Up (p. 92)
Lack of hip mobility in squats » Poor performance; lower-back, knee, and hip issues	Hip Strength & Mobility (p. 58) · Knee Strength (p. 60) · Resistance Athlete's Strength, Mobility, Flexibility & Balance (p. 68) · Overall Hip Flexibility (p. 76) · Adductor & Hamstring Flexibility (p. 77) · Glute, Hip Flexor & Quadricep Flexibility (p. 78)
Shoulder inflexibility, especially in an overhead press » Underdevelopment of upper back muscles; overuse of chest muscles; rotator cuff and shoulder issues	Total Upper-Body Strength (p. 61) · Shoulder Strength (p. 62) · Muscular Imbalance Correction (p. 64) · Shoulder Flexibility (p. 80) · Warm-Up for Healthy Shoulders (p. 94)
Lack of spinal mobility » Back and spine issues	Muscular Imbalance Correction (p. 64) · Total Spine Mobility (p. 82) · Full-Body Flexibility & Mobility (p. 84)
Lack of ankle mobility » Knee pain; instability	Balance Strength (p. 53) · Balance for Hips, Ankles, Knees & Core (p. 56) · Ankle Stability (p. 57) · Foot & Ankle Mobility (p. 81)

MUSCLE WEAKNESS

The most common weaknesses present in weight lifters can be grouped into one of two categories: (1) muscular imbalances, and (2) lack of muscle activation.

A muscular imbalance refers to a disproportionate amount of strength between two muscle groups. In weight-training terms, this typically means exercising certain muscle groups more than others. All of us have muscular imbalances, and we unknowingly reinforce these imbalances on a daily basis, both in our workouts *and* when we are not exercising. Learning about your imbalances and addressing them with the appropriate exercises can reduce your risk of injury, improve your performance, and ensure your longevity.

A lack of muscle activation is the other main source of muscular weakness in weight-training athletes. This term goes by a lot of phrases, but whether you say "mind-body awareness," "motor control," or "getting your muscles to turn on," the meaning is generally the same: being able to use a given muscle appropriately during an exercise. **Here are some common areas of muscular imbalances and muscle activation issues:**

SHOULDERS

Often the muscles of the front of the torso and shoulders are strong, but the muscles in the back are weak. Excess pushing exercises (push-ups, bench presses, etc.) and not enough pulling or scapular strength work (pull-ups, rows, rear-deltoid strengtheners, etc.) causes this imbalance, and poor muscle activation in the pulling muscles and scapular stabilizers reinforces the imbalance.

WEAKNESS » SYMPTOM	BUILD YOUR PRACTICE WITH THESE WORKOUTS
Weak pulling muscles/ scapular stabilizers » Overactive pushing muscles; shoulder impingement; rotator cuff issues; biceps tears	Total Upper-Body Strength (p. 61) · Shoulder Strength (p. 62) · Shoulder Flexibility (p. 80) · Warm-Up for Healthy Shoulders (p. 94)

HIPS

Many weight lifters assume they're properly targeting their glutes, but they are really just targeting their quadriceps and lower back. Poor glute activation even throws your posture out of balance, which can cause shoulder issues. Improving glute activation helps to relieve pressure on the knees and lower back, strengthen the hips, improve performance, and greatly prevent injury.

WEAKNESS » SYMPTOM	BUILD YOUR PRACTICE WITH THESE WORKOUTS
Inactive or weak glutes; overactive quadriceps » Knee, back, hip, and shoulder issues	Balance Strength (p. 53) · No-Impact Lower-Body Endurance (p. 54) · Balance for Hips, Ankles, Knees & Core (p. 56) · Knee Strength (p. 60) · Muscular Imbalance Correction (p. 64) · Resistance Athlete's Strength, Mobility, Flexibility & Balance (p. 68) · All-Purpose Warm-Up to Prevent Joint Pain During Workouts (p. 88) · Compound Strength Movement Warm-Up (p. 92)

CORE

Your core is the area from your mid-thighs all the way up to your ribs. Many weight lifters have a strong rectus abdominis (six-pack) but lack comprehensive core strength. Inactive abdominals during lifting workouts leads to significant back issues. An inactive core cannot stabilize the spine. You will have limited performance and place additional stress on the knees. It also results in a dramatic imbalance between the front (abdomen) and back (erector spinae) of your lower torso, placing a significant burden on the lower back. This causes pain and can lead to more serious back issues over time. (I've spoken to many former athletes who have had to give up what they're doing entirely because of nagging issues that went unaddressed. Don't be like them!)

WEAKNESS » SYMPTOM	BUILD YOUR PRACTICE WITH THESE WORKOUTS
Lack of overall core strength; poor spinal strength and mobility; weak pelvic floor and hips » Back, hip, and knee issues	Total Core Strength (p. 52) · Balance Strength (p. 53) · Balance for Hips, Ankles, Knees & Core (p. 56) · Muscular Imbalance Correction (p. 64) · All-Purpose Warm-Up to Prevent Joint Pain During Workouts (p. 88) · Compound Strength Movement Warm-Up (p. 92)

TRAINING GAPS

Using yoga to address the training gaps of traditional strength training not only improves your lifting—it also dramatically improves your performance in all of your physical activities.

BREATH WORK, BODY AWARENESS & MINDFULNESS

Most of us don't consciously think about our breathing. It's only when something else brings our attention to our breathing that we even think about it. But working on your breathing actually significantly improves your lifting. Breathing helps pump freshly oxygenated blood through your body, eliminates cellular waste, and prevents dangerous rises in blood pressure. It enables you to maintain focus and continue going strong during those longer sets, but it also helps you avoid dizziness and passing out, which can undoubtedly ruin a day at the gym.

Yoga places a huge emphasis on breathing, which is invaluable for addressing some of the slower, more mindful aspects of fitness that can dramatically improve overall physical fitness and well being. (For direct focus on improving your breathing, check out "Breath Work with Guest Coach Brian Mackenzie" on page 16.)

While practicing your breathing in conjunction with movement, you begin to realize the effect breathing has on your body. Breathing can help you work deeper into your flexibility by helping to calm your sympathetic nervous system. You also gain a greater awareness of the impact that breathing has on your ability to remain in control over your body and to keep pushing when you feel tired. This is great for when you're trying to hit those last few reps and are struggling both mentally and physically. Reestablishing control over yourself by checking in on your breathing is extremely helpful in situations like these. In just a few weeks of consistent yoga practice, breathing properly should carry over to your weight training, and you'll notice that your improved breathing is also improving your performance in your resistance training.

This is also how mindfulness is developed. Continuous movement is one thing, but when you're holding a posture for 30, 45, or 60 seconds—that's when you have enough time to really focus on body awareness. Recommitting your mental focus to proper technique, breathing to support subtle changes in your body, and noticing the effects of these subtle changes all help to develop mindfulness. Mindfulness strengthens you mentally by improving your ability to focus, and who wouldn't want more of that?

For better breathing and body awareness, build your practice with this workout.	Postures to Practice Diaphragmatic Breathing (p. 17)

ISOMETRIC TRAINING

Weight lifting is dynamic; you're constantly moving and doing reps. Aside from Abs Day when you do a few sets of planks, how often are you using isometric strength?

Isometric exercises are nonmoving exercises, during which the length of the target muscles remains mostly the same, and the affected joints don't move. The most well-known example is a plank, but there are so many other isometric exercises, and they don't just have to target your abs. Although the movement of transitioning *between* the postures is part of yoga, the yoga poses themselves are isometric exercises.

Isometric strengthening is important because it helps to build joint stability and improve muscular performance. The more isometric strength you have, the greater your overall strength potential.

Another added bonus of isometric exercise is that it's perfect for a warm-up. Holding postures for even 15 seconds is a great way to flush blood into the targeted muscles, improving the muscle activation of those areas and "turning on" those muscles for exercise.

For a focus on isometric training, build your practice with these workouts.	All of them! Every workout and posture in the book has elements of isometric training.

FLEXIBILITY & MOBILITY TRAINING

Aside from the stretching routines you *might* do (but are probably skipping) before and after your workout, how often are you actually focusing on your flexibility? Ideally, your flexibility training involves much more than just stretching. While stretching is certainly helpful, the benefits are mostly temporary.

In order to create lasting improvement, we want to practice exercises that demand us to combine strength with flexibility, and we need to push the limits of our maximum range of motion while doing it. This is why practicing yoga with an emphasis on strength and proper muscle activation is so helpful. You'll learn exactly which muscles to focus on engaging for each posture in the poses section of this book.

Yoga in particular focuses on bringing you to your end range of motion, and the right instructional cues will then train you to build strength there. For example, the High Lunge (p. 130) is a basic lunge position which allows you to simultaneously build strength and mobility. As you work deeper into the posture, eventually you reach a point where you can go no deeper while safely maintaining proper technique, but you'll continue to use your strength to hold the position. This is where strength at end range of motion occurs. Adding this training to your workouts dramatically improves muscular performance.

For flexibility and mobility training, build your practice with these workouts.	All of them! Every workout and posture in the book has elements of mobility improvement.

BALANCE TRAINING

Balance is remaining steady, especially in compromised or unsteady positions, such as remaining stable in one-sided exercises or exercises where your weight is on one leg, or if you're standing on an unsteady surface. In the context of yoga, balance training generally refers specifically to practicing stability while standing on one foot while executing a specific posture with your body.

Balance is part skill and part strength. It is a skill in that balancing is a coordination we develop with practice and

focus, but it is also strength in that our bodies have to develop the strength and mobility required for balance.

Balance work is incredibly useful for your ankles, knees, and hips. It's one of the most effective forms of exercise to prevent injury in these areas. Regularly practicing your balance with the appropriate exercise is often enough to prevent chronic knee and back pain because it's *that effective* at strengthening the weaknesses that cause those issues to begin with. The more balance work you can do, the more you're doing to maintain and improve the overall strength and stability of your lower body.

For balance training, build your practice with these workouts.	Total Core Strength (p. 52) · Balance Strength (p. 53) · Balance for Hips, Ankles, Knees & Core (p. 56) · Ankle Stability (p. 57) · Hip Strength & Mobility (p. 58) · Knee Strength (p. 60) · Foot & Ankle Mobility (p. 81) · All-Purpose Warm-Up to Prevent Joint Pain During Workouts (p. 88)

RECOVERY & RESTORATIVE WORK

Your body only grows stronger through recovery. The act of lifting weights actually breaks down your muscle fibers, and the restorative process—your body's response to the breaking down of muscle fibers—helps to facilitate the recovery process that repairs (i.e. grows) muscle. If you are not actively engaged in activities to help assist this process, you are not only delaying recovery, but you are also inhibiting your strength progress.

Yoga helps with recovery and restoration in three ways:

1. The restorative stretches allow your muscles to relax, to release tension, to lengthen, and to recover.

2. The active recovery process of stretching (as opposed to sitting and doing nothing) also helps to flush dead tissue from broken-down muscle fibers and speeds along recovery.

3. The slow, controlled breathing practiced while doing yoga helps to activate the body's parasympathetic nervous response, sending your body into a state of "rest and digest," during which your body focuses on repairing and building your body back up.

What's really cool about these benefits? You'll notice them *immediately*—not two months from now, not one month from now, but immediately. Taking the time to practice yoga with an emphasis on recovery, stretching, and breathing allows you to return to your workouts feeling stronger and better rested. When you're stretched, your joints feel better and your movement feels smoother, and you're able to push yourself harder in your workouts.

For recovery training, build your practice with these workouts and poses.

Workouts: Overall Hip Flexibility (p. 76) · Adductor & Hamstring Flexibility (p. 77) · Glute, Hip Flexor & Quadricep Flexibility (p. 78) · Shoulder Flexibility (p. 80) · Foot & Ankle Mobility (p. 81) · Total Spine Mobility (p. 82) · Full-Body Flexibility & Mobility (p. 84)

Poses: Bridge: Supported on Block (p. 111) · Child's Pose (p. 116) · Downdog: On Wall (p. 123) · Frog (p. 124) · Lizard (p. 134) · Pigeon (p. 138) · Standing Sidebend: On Wall (p. 159) · Reclined Strap Stretches (p. 142) · Thread the Needle (p. 160) · Triangle: Supported on Block (p. 165) · Wide-Legged Forward Fold (p. 170)

PAIN POINTS

You probably have certain problem areas that limit your workouts. For the more common pain points, yoga can be an effective way to not only manage the symptoms, but also to solve their root causes. Let's look at typical injuries, their causes, and the weaknesses that need to be addressed to fix them. Yoga is perfect for prevention, so even if you don't have the injury yet, you can start working on them today to lower the risk of the injury occurring. Use the table to find the pain points that are keeping you from getting stronger. Find the corresponding workouts or poses to begin improving.

AREA	SPECIFIC INJURY OR ISSUE	CAUSES	CORRECTIVE AREAS OF FOCUS	BUILD YOUR PRACTICE WITH THESE WORKOUTS AND POSES
FEET/ ANKLES	**Injuries:** Achilles tendinitis; Achilles tendon rupture; plantar fasciitis **Pains and discomforts:** Achilles tightness; calf strain; general feet pain	Lack of ankle strength Lack of ankle mobility Improper technique Flat feet or weak arches	Ankle mobility Ankle strength Arch strength Balance	**Workouts:** Balance Strength (p. 53) · Balance for Hips, Ankles, Knees & Core (p. 56) · Ankle Stability (p. 57) · Knee Strength (p. 60) · Resistance Athlete's Strength, Mobility, Flexibility & Balance (p. 68) · Foot & Ankle Mobility (p. 81) **Poses:** Airplane (p. 104) · Chair (p. 114) · Downdog (p. 122), High Lunge (p. 130) · Tree (p. 162) · Warrior 1 (p. 166) · Warrior 2 (p. 168) · Wide-Legged Forward Fold (p. 170)
KNEES	**Injuries:** Meniscus/ MCL tear; patellar tendinitis **Pains and discomforts:** General knee pain during/after exercise; knee clicking during squats, lunges, or dead lifts	Lack of hip, ankle, and core strength and stability Lack of hip and ankle mobility	Ankle mobility Ankle strength Balance Core strength General recovery stretching to prevent overtraining Hip strength Hip mobility	**Workouts:** Total Core Strength (p. 52) · Balance Strength (p. 53) · No-Impact Lower-Body Endurance (p. 54) · Balance for Hips, Ankles, Knees & Core (p. 56) · Ankle Stability (p. 57) · Hip Strength & Mobility (p. 58) · Knee Strength (p. 60) · Muscular Imbalance Correction (p. 64) · Overall Hip Flexibility (p. 76) · Adductor & Hamstring Flexibility (p. 77) · Glute, Hip Flexor & Quadricep Flexibility (p. 78) · Foot & Ankle Mobility (p. 81) · All-Purpose Warm-Up to Prevent Joint Pain During Workouts (p. 88) · Compound Strength Movement Warm-Up (p. 92) · Knee Soreness Relief (p. 95) **Poses:** Airplane (p. 104) · Boat (p. 108) · Bridge (p. 110) · Chair (p. 114) · Cobra (p. 118) · Dolphin (p. 120) · Downdog (p. 122) · Frog (p. 124) · Full Locust (p. 126) · High Lunge (p. 130) · Horse (p. 132) · Lizard (p. 134) · Pigeon (p. 138) · Pyramid (p. 140) · Reclined Strap Stretches (p. 142) · Side Plank (p. 152) · Standing Bow (p. 156) · Tree (p. 162) · Triangle (p. 164) · Warrior 2 (p. 168) · Wide-Legged Forward Fold (p. 170)

AREA	SPECIFIC INJURY OR ISSUE	CAUSES	CORRECTIVE AREAS OF FOCUS	BUILD YOUR PRACTICE WITH THESE WORKOUTS AND POSES
LOWER BACK	**Injuries:** Herniated discs; slipped discs; spinal fusion surgery **Pains and discomforts:** Lack of thoracic mobility (rotating spine from side to side); neck pain; general lower-back pain	Lack of core and hip strength Lack of hip and spine mobility	Balance Core strength Hip mobility Hip strength Posture Spinal mobility	**Workouts:** Total Core Strength (p. 52) · Balance Strength (p. 53) · Hip Strength & Mobility (p. 58) · Muscular Imbalance Correction (p. 64) · Overall Hip Flexibility (p. 76) · Total Spine Mobility (p. 82) · All-Purpose Warm-Up to Prevent Joint Pain During Workouts (p. 88) · Compound Strength Movement Warm-Up (p. 92) · Back Pain Relief (p. 98) · Total Spine Relief (p. 99) **Poses:** Airplane (p. 104) · Boat (p. 108) · Bridge (p. 110) · Chair (p. 114) · Child's Pose (p. 116) · Frog (p. 124) · Full Locust (p. 126) · Horse (p. 132) · Lizard (p. 134) · Pigeon (p. 138) · Reclined Strap Stretches (p. 142) · Reclined Twist (p. 144) · Side Plank (p. 152) · Standing Backbend (p. 154) · Standing Side Bend (p. 158) · Tree (p. 162)
MIDDLE AND UPPER BACK	**Injuries:** Herniated discs; spondylitis **Pains and discomforts:** Middle- and upper-back pain and stiffness	Lack of thoracic mobility (rotating from side to side) Poor posture Upper-back weakness Core weakness	Core strength Posture Spinal mobility Spinal strength	**Workouts:** Total Core Strength (p. 52) · Balance Strength (p. 53) · Total Upper-Body Strength (p. 61) · Shoulder Strength (p. 62) · Shoulder Flexibility (p. 80) · Total Spine Mobility (p. 82) · Warm-Up For Healthy Shoulders (p. 94) · Back Pain Relief (p. 98) · Total Spine Relief (p. 99) **Poses:** Boat (p. 108) · Bridge (p. 110) · Child's Pose (p. 116) · Cobra (p. 118) · Dolphin (p. 120) · Downdog (p. 122) · Full Locust (p. 126) · Reclined Twist (p. 144) · Seated Twist (p. 148) · Side Angle (p. 150) · Standing Back Bend (p. 154) · Standing Bow (p. 156) · Standing Side Bend (p. 158) · Thread the Needle (p. 160) · Tree (p. 162) · Wide-Legged Forward Fold (p. 170)
HEAD AND NECK	**Injuries:** Cervical radiculopathy; herniated discs; cervical spondylosis **Pains and discomforts:** General neck pain; pain when turning head from side to side; limited range of motion	Lack of cervical mobility Poor posture General neck weakness	Core strength Hip mobility Hip strength Posture Upper-back strength	**Workouts:** Total Core Strength (p. 52) · Balance Strength (p. 53) · Balance for Hips, Ankles, Knees & Core (p. 56) · Knee Strength (p. 60) · Total Upper-Body Strength (p. 61) · Shoulder Strength (p. 62) · Muscular Imbalance Correction (p. 64) · Resistance Athlete's Strength, Mobility, Flexibility & Balance (p. 68) · Full-Body Strength, Mobility & Injury Prevention (p. 72) · Overall Hip Flexibility (p. 76) · Adductor & Hamstring Flexibility (p. 77) · Glute, Hip Flexor & Quadricep Flexibility (p. 78) · Shoulder Flexibility (p. 80) · Total Spine Mobility (p. 82) · Full-Body Flexibility & Mobility (p. 84) · Compound Strength Movement Warm-Up (p. 92) · Warm-Up For Healthy Shoulders (p. 94) · Back Pain Relief (p. 98) · Total Spine Relief (p. 99) **Poses:** Boat (p. 108) · Child's Pose (p. 116) · Cobra (p. 118) · Dolphin (p. 120) · Downdog (p. 122) · Full Locust (p. 126) · Seated Twist (p. 148) · Side Angle (p. 150) · Standing Backbend (p. 154) · Standing Sidebend (p. 158) · Tree (p. 162) · Warrior 2 (p. 168)

AREA	SPECIFIC INJURY OR ISSUE	CAUSES	CORRECTIVE AREAS OF FOCUS	BUILD YOUR PRACTICE WITH THESE WORKOUTS AND POSES
SHOULDERS	**Injuries:** Rotator cuff tear; biceps tear; shoulder impingement **Pains and discomforts:** General shoulder pain	Lack of shoulder mobility Lack of scapular stabilizing strength Poor posture	Scapular stability Shoulder mobility	**Workouts:** Total Upper-Body Strength (p. 61) · Shoulder Strength (p. 62) · Resistance Athlete's Strength, Mobility, Flexibility & Balance (p. 68) · Shoulder Flexibility (p. 80) · Total Spine Mobility (p. 82) · Warm-Up For Healthy Shoulders (p. 94) · Upper-Body & Shoulder Soreness Relief (p. 96) **Poses:** Airplane: Warrior 3 (p. 105) · Child's Pose (p. 116) · Cobra (p. 118) · Dolphin (p. 120) · Downdog (p. 122) · Full Locust (p. 126) · Side Angle (p. 150) · Side Plank (p. 152) · Standing Backbend (p. 154) · Standing Sidebend (p. 158) · Thread the Needle (p. 160) · Tree (p. 162) · Triangle (p. 164) · Wide-Legged Forward Fold: With Strap and Twist (p. 171)

HOW TO PRACTICE YOGA WHEN YOU HAVE PAIN POINTS

While some yoga postures may be helpful, I do not recommend yoga as an alternative to physical therapy. To ensure you are doing the appropriate exercises to facilitate recovery, you should find a licensed physical therapist who focuses on exercise-based rehabilitation.

As a general rule of thumb: If it hurts, don't do it. While injured or recovering from injury, some of these postures will be accessible, while others will not. Discomfort is okay, but avoid sharp or shooting pain. These guidelines are meant to address minor injuries, and they should not be used to replace the advice of a physical therapist or an orthopedic doctor. Every situation is unique, so make sure you have a proper conversation with a licensed medical professional before exercising with a significant injury.

For lower-body injuries: Avoid any weight-bearing or standing postures. This means that you should not do any exercises where you are placing weight on the affected leg. Focus on non-weight-bearing exercises instead.

For back injuries: Depending on the severity of the injury, generally you will want to stay active to facilitate recovery. Just make sure that the exercises are not causing you any pain. Keep range of motion limited; avoid deep forward folds, twists, or backbends.

For upper-body injuries: Many of the postures will be accessible, but you may have to modify how you use your hands. For example, if you have a shoulder injury, you're welcome to practice lunge-like yoga postures, but you should keep your arms relaxed at your sides instead of lifting them overhead.

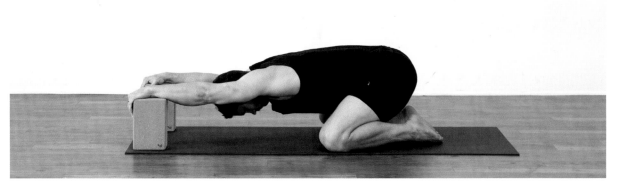

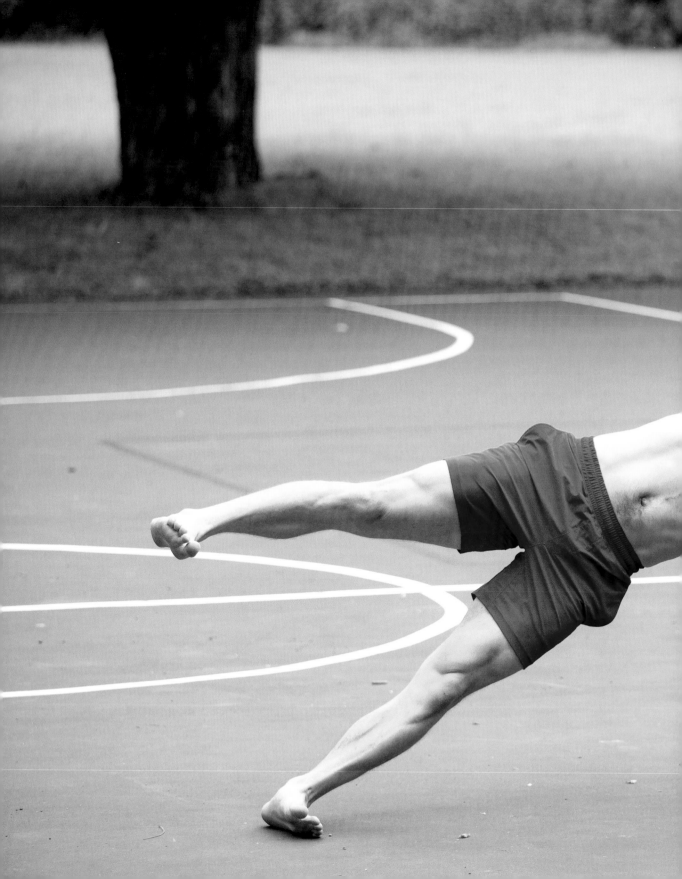

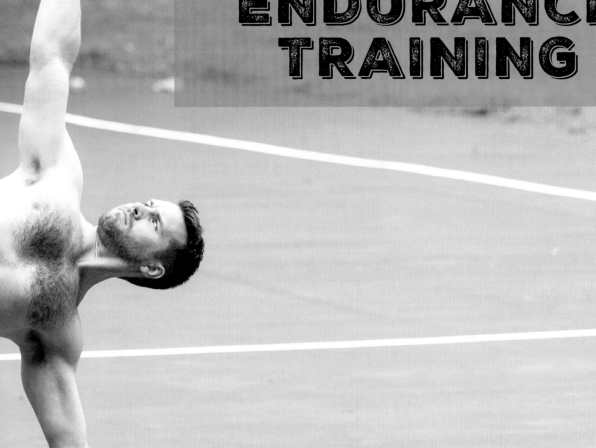

CHAPTER 3 »
YOGA FOR ENDURANCE TRAINING

THE ENDURANCE ATHLETE

Endurance athletes typically have great levels of endurance and cardiovascular abilities, but because the nature of their training requires such repetitive movement, they inevitably miss out on movements and exercises that could dramatically improve their performance. They also contribute to existing imbalances that can eventually lead to injury, if unchecked. In this section, you'll learn how yoga can help endurance athletes improve their performance and reduce their risk of injury. Adding consistent yoga to your weekly training can be done with relatively little time and effort, and the benefits of doing so will be realized in just a few workouts—maybe even less.

USING THIS CHAPTER

To help you understand common weaknesses of endurance athletes, we'll explore common injuries, problem areas, and training gaps, and explain how yoga can help address each of these directly. Alongside an overview of these items, each specific topic covered directs you to routines or specific postures that will help you address your goals. (For example, if we are discussing a lack of strength training, we include a routine you can use to develop strength.) Choose from the recommended workouts for your goals, and aim to get in about six workouts per week.

CONSISTENCY & RESULTS

If you can do 60 minutes of yoga per week, you should notice the results within just four weeks—and most likely, even sooner. Your movement will feel smoother, your joints will feel better, and you won't take as long to recover. You need to keep it up to continue to notice the results. If you stop doing yoga, those noticeable improvements will start to go away within weeks.

HOW CAN YOGA HELP WITH ENDURANCE TRAINING

Your training probably has predictable gaps and common pain points. Here's an overview of what you have to look forward to with a targeted and consistent yoga practice.

Decrease risk of preventable injuries, aches, and pains:

- Fix overtraining injuries from excessive training
- Build muscular endurance, without as much stress on the joints
- Use recovery training to speed up recovery time and prevent overtraining injury

Increase strength in commonly weak areas:

- Improve muscle efficiency and overall strength; increase bone density to lower risk of injury
- Correct muscular imbalances to reduce strain on joints, ligaments, and tendons

Increase mobility and flexibility:

- Improve movement efficiency
- Speed up recovery time
- Decrease overall risk of injury

Improve breathing:

- Improve posture and overall movement technique, which helps to decrease injury
- Increase endurance capacity
- Improve cardiovascular ability

Increase mindfulness:

- Enhance ability to focus and power through difficult moments
- Improve ability to check in with your body and make necessary adjustments

ENDURANCE TRAINING
WITH GUEST COACH NICK BARE

Over the course of the past 10 years, I've experimented with all types and styles of physical training. While serving a contract with the US Army as an Infantry Officer, I learned how to suffer through brutal training exercises and military schools. I have a background in strength and conditioning that I focused on while earning my degree in nutrition during my college years, and today I lean more toward endurance sports.

I've trained for and completed triathlons (Ironman distance), and multiple marathons, and am now moving into the ultra-marathon distance scene—it's an addicting way to train. I find the solitude during aerobic endurance training is a very powerful tool, not only for the body, but more importantly for the mind. It has very similar benefits to incorporating yoga into your fitness routine, which is why I like to include it in my weekly programming.

After many years of exercising, I've learned how to be very conscious of my body and self-aware of how I'm feeling, recovering, and progressing through training cycles. Entering the world of endurance sports taught me many things that quickly humbled me, but one of those observations was my lack of mobility and flexibility. I had a thorough understanding of the importance of strength training in endurance; however, the necessity of mobility to these extremes was brand new.

Prior to endurance sports, if lack of mobility was ever an issue, I would just modify an exercise in order to get a similar benefit, which is one of the reasons I forever avoided the squat snatch. However, while training for my first triathlon, I quickly learned the necessity of proper mobility and how yoga could help me reach my fitness goals. Running always seemed second nature to me, which is probably due to the miles we totaled in the army. However, swimming and cycling were completely out of my comfort zone. My first time sitting on a time-trial bike proved how tight my hamstrings and hips were. My inability to use any range of motion with my shoulders prevented me from reaching an aerodynamic position on the bike. What did I do? I started incorporating yoga positions into my weekly routine. This wasn't the first time

I started practicing yoga, though. A few years prior, while diving into the world of CrossFit, I realized the importance of mobility—it was always a weakness of mine.

In order to get into a more aerodynamic position on the bike, which would allow me to ride faster in a more efficient fit, I learned how to use poses such as pigeon, lizard, child's pose, pyramid, downdog, dolphin, thread the needle, and high lunge to improve mobility. As I incorporated yoga into my morning routine, I also realized it was helping with my swim training. After years of weight lifting and a lack of shoulder mobility, my stroke was naturally inefficient. I wasn't able to get a high elbow position for an effective catch, but that slowly started to improve with more yoga poses targeting upper-body mobility. All of the time I spent running, swimming, and cycling was now starting to become more effective and efficient because these yoga poses were making huge improvements to my mobility.

Not only has yoga helped me become more aerodynamic and efficient in aspects of endurance training, it has also helped with the overuse of repetitive movements. During my third marathon build, which was shortly after my first Ironman prep, I developed overuse symptoms in my left knee, hips, and ankles. Passive and active poses have helped fix the overuse issues and prevent new ones. Over the past couple years, yoga has been a staple in my routine to avoid injuries and improve efficiencies for endurance training. Yoga for me is not about going to classes or studios (which I'm not by any means against), but rather about preworkout mobility and activation, as well as nighttime recovery. I do these movements in the comfort of my home, and they allow me to train harder and smarter in everything I do.

WEAKNESSES

As an endurance athlete, you have great levels of fitness relative to your discipline of choice (running, cycling, swimming, etc.), but because of your training, you unknowingly create and reinforce imbalances. You may also omit strength in areas not directly addressed by your endurance training, which, ironically, hurts you as an endurance athlete. In this section, we'll point out endurance athlete–specific weaknesses and training gaps, and discuss how yoga can help with issues like runner's knee, lower-back pain, overtraining symptoms, and more.

LACK OF FLEXIBILITY & MOBILITY

Endurance athletes do not often focus on flexibility, and this leads to muscle tightness that can cause discomfort during your workouts and worse, lead to injuries or imbalances that force you to stop training. Runners in particular complain about hamstring tightness, cyclists have tight hip flexors, and nearly every endurance athlete has had a sore back at some point. There is a general tightening of muscles that occurs following a workout. Flexibility training helps alleviate this tightness on a short-term basis; however, the more frequently you can include flexibility in your training routine (at least three times weekly), and to the extent you can combine flexibility *and* strength (to form mobility), the less overall muscle tightness you'll experience.

Mobility refers to strength within flexibility. For endurance athletes, this allows you to more effectively build strength in range of motion, addressing muscular imbalances that can hinder performance and increase risk of preventable injury. Generally speaking, if you can improve your mobility, you can address many of the symptoms that cause excessive soreness—which, if unchecked, can lead to chronic pain or injury—to begin with.

Endurance athletes should focus on flexibility to increase potential mobility, while also promoting recovery and relieving soreness from workouts. Mobility training helps you lock in your flexibility and see more noticeable improvements in your overall performance. You'll need both in order to succeed. **If you have any of the issues below, consider the recommended routines:**

INFLEXIBILITY » SYMPTOM	BUILD YOUR PRACTICE WITH THESE WORKOUTS
Hamstring/adductor tightness » Lower-back, knee, or hip pain	Hip Strength & Mobility (p. 58) · Knee Strength (p. 60) · Muscular Imbalance Correction (p. 64) · Runner's Strength, Flexibility & Balance (p. 66) · Overall Hip Flexibility (p. 76) · Adductor & Hamstring Flexibility (p. 77) · Knee Soreness Relief (p. 95)
Quadriceps and hip flexors tightness » Knee, back, or hip pain	Hip Strength & Mobility (p. 58) · Knee Strength (p. 60) · Runner's Strength, Flexibility & Balance (p. 66) · Endurance Athlete's Strength, Mobility, Flexibility & Balance (p. 70) · Overall Hip Flexibility (p. 76) · Glute, Hip Flexor & Quadricep Flexibility (p. 78) · Knee Soreness Relief (p. 95)
Glute tightness » Knee, hip, or back pain	Overall Hip Flexibility (p. 76) · Glute, Hip Flexor & Quadricep Flexibility (p. 78)
Ankle tightness » Ankle, foot, knee, or back pain	Foot & Ankle Mobility (p. 81) · Knee Soreness Relief (p. 95)
Back tightness » Back, neck, shoulder, hip, or knee pain	Total Core Strength (p. 52) · Balance Strength (p. 53) · Hip Strength & Mobility (p. 58) · Overall Hip Flexibility (p. 76) · Adductor & Hamstring Flexibility (p. 77) · Glute, Hip Flexor & Quadricep Flexibility (p. 78) · Total Spine Mobility (p. 82) · All-Purpose Warm-Up to Prevent Joint Pain During Workouts (p. 88) · Runner's Warm-Up (p. 91) · Endurance Athlete's Warm-Up (p. 90) · Upper-Body & Shoulder Soreness Relief (p. 96) · Back Pain Relief (p. 98) · Total Spine Relief (p. 99)
Shoulder tightness » Shoulder, neck, or back pain	Shoulder Flexibility (p. 80) · Total Spine Mobility (p. 82) · Upper-Body & Shoulder Soreness Relief (p. 96)

MUSCLE WEAKNESS

A lack of overall strength puts you at a higher risk of injury and increases the strain on your joints. Running, swimming, and other forms of endurance training build endurance, but that's not the same thing as strength. Strength is necessary to keep your joints strong, improve your performance, and avoid injury. Although we often associate joint pain with muscle tightness, overall muscle weakness is also a common cause. It is vital to address not only the weak muscles in question, but also to build strength in the antagonist (opposing) muscle groups.

Muscular imbalances are caused by the repetitive movements involved in endurance sports. The muscles targeted during endurance training workouts are well conditioned, but the opposing muscle groups (the antagonists) are weak. These imbalances leave the athlete at a higher risk of injury. You should be sure to add the appropriate exercises to your weekly routines both to build a baseline level of strength for these neglected areas and also to counter your endurance training. Your daily activities (especially sitting) also have an impact on imbalances. Sitting for four or more hours per day can tighten your hips and shoulders, weaken your core, and limit overall mobility. These imbalances carry over into your workouts, so it's important to do the right mobility exercises to undo this inactivity. Endurance athletes should focus on a full-body approach to correct imbalances.

UPPER BODY

Endurance athletes need the strength to hold their upper bodies in a strong, upright position to ensure optimal breathing. Without that strength in the chest, shoulders, and upper back, they could find themselves performing at lower levels than expected. Working on upper-body strength while reinforcing good posture can dramatically improve performance.

WEAKNESS » SYMPTOM	BUILD YOUR PRACTICE WITH THESE WORKOUTS
Poor upper-body strength » Improper posture; decreased breathing efficiency; high risk of injury due to anatomically incorrect movement	Total Core Strength (p. 52) · Total Upper-Body Strength (p. 61) · Shoulder Strength (p. 62)

CORE

Endurance athletes may have strength in certain areas of the core, but their usual training involves movements that occur in the sagittal plane—moving forward or backward in a straight line—and not enough movements that involve twisting (transverse plane) or side-to-side (frontal/coronal plane) motions. Including these types of movements increases overall core strength, but more importantly, it decreases your risk of injury significantly.

WEAKNESS » SYMPTOM	BUILD YOUR PRACTICE WITH THESE WORKOUTS
Poor core strength » Hip, back, and knee issues; suboptimal overall performance	Total Core Strength (p. 52) · Balance Strength (p. 53) · Balance for Hips, Ankles, Knees & Core (p. 56) · Total Upper-Body Strength (p. 61) · Muscular Imbalance Correction (p. 64) · Transverse & Frontal Plane Movements (p.65) · Full-Body Strength, Mobility & Injury Prevention (p. 72)

HIPS & LOWER BODY

Most endurance athletes are quadriceps dominant and lack strength in the glutes. This is mainly due to a lack of exercise that specifically addresses the posterior chain. This leads to issues like IT band syndrome or runner's knee. It even throws your posture out of balance, which can cause shoulder issues. Strengthening the hips (and the glutes in particular) with the targeted yoga poses in this book enables you to train more frequently with a lower risk of injury, decreases joint pain or joint stiffness during and after your workouts, and helps to support bone density for increased longevity.

WEAKNESS » SYMPTOM	BUILD YOUR PRACTICE WITH THESE WORKOUTS
Strong quadriceps, weak glutes » Knee, back, hip, and shoulder issues **Poor lower-body strength; continuous joint strain »** Pain in lower body joints and spine	Balance Strength (p. 53) · No-Impact Lower-Body Endurance (p. 54) · Balance for Hips, Ankles, Knees & Core (p. 56) · Hip Strength & Mobility (p. 58) · Knee Strength (p. 60) · Muscular Imbalance Correction (p. 64) · Runner's Strength, Flexibility & Balance (p. 66)

TRAINING GAPS

When it comes to additional training, endurance athletes can best benefit from workouts that fill the gaps of their existing endurance training. This is important to improve performance, but is perhaps even more important as a means of avoiding preventable injuries. This section provides detailed information on the most significant training gaps of the typical endurance athlete, as well as postures and routines that will directly fill these gaps.

STRENGTH TRAINING

Building strength is incredibly important to the endurance athlete. Endurance does not equal muscular strength, and this is what you need in order to support your joints, prevent injury, and maintain bone density. Effective strength training also includes a mobility component. That's why it's important to work on improving the depth of your exercises (i.e. how deep you can go into a squat or lunge) while maintaining strength. This makes yoga an ideal strength-training solution.

You don't need anything other than your body to start building strength, and with the right yoga postures, you can adequately build strength to complement your endurance training and reduce your risk of injury. The important thing to remember is you want to push yourself to the point of failure to experience noticeable strength gains, so be sure to challenge yourself.

For better full-body strength, build your practice with these workouts.	Total Core Strength (p. 52) · Balance Strength (p. 53) · No-Impact Lower-Body Endurance (p. 54) · Total Upper-Body Strength (p. 61) · Muscular Imbalance Correction (p. 64) · Runner's Strength, Flexibility & Balance (p. 66) · Endurance Athlete's Strength, Mobility, Flexibility & Balance (p. 70) · Full-Body Strength, Mobility & Injury Prevention (p. 72)

BREATH WORK

The ability to maintain your breathing is incredibly important to performing your best in endurance training. Training your breathing to be as efficient as possible helps you to maintain a moderately intense level of exercise for a longer period of time. The emphasis on breathing found in yoga is invaluable for addressing some of the slower, more mindful aspects of fitness that can dramatically improve overall physical fitness and wellbeing. Practicing yoga regularly helps to develop breath awareness, and understand the relationship between your body and your breath (if you can maintain control over your breathing, you can maintain control over your body), and allows you to practice using your breath to push your body through physical discomfort. The breathing emphasized in yoga is called "diaphragmatic breathing" (p. 16). Diaphragmatic breathing helps you fully use your diaphragm to make your breathing as effective and efficient as possible. This breathing even helps you maintain the integrity of your posture, ensuring your hips, core, and shoulders remain in proper alignment. This improves your performance, reduces injury and strain on your joints, and just makes movement feel better.

The more you can practice this breathing during yoga, the more it will carry over into your endurance workouts. Slowing things down to practice simultaneous awareness of your breath and body helps to develop mindfulness. This allows you to better check in with your body and make needed adjustments, whether that's powering through a difficult section of a course or remembering to breathe when you're feeling tired.

One other big benefit of practicing breath awareness while doing yoga is noticing that your breathing enables you to keep going. Very generally speaking, as long as you can maintain control over your breathing, you can continue to push yourself to remain in the posture for the required hold time.

This carries over into your endurance training, as well. When you're pushing yourself to maintain a difficult pace or feel yourself starting to become anxious, remembering to breathe can help you stay in control and maintain your composure. You remember that as long as you can continue to breathe, you can keep your body in check and keep pushing forward.

For better breath work, build your practice with these workouts.	Postures to Practice Diaphragmatic Breathing (p. 17) · Total Core Strength (p. 52) · Full-Body Flexibility & Mobility (p. 84) · Full-Body Restoration (p. 100)

ISOMETRIC & SLOWER-MOVING EXERCISE

There is no slow, controlled movement in endurance training, and it is exactly these slower or nonmoving elements that can fill the strength and mobility gaps of your fitness. Isometrics and slow movement won't simulate a race, but they do help you in other ways:

- **Build strength in new ways.** By changing the speed (tempo) of your exercises, you can improve your overall strength when compared to exercising at one speed.

- **Develop joint stability and foundational strength.** Isometrics are fantastic for developing joint strength stability. They also allow you to build strength that forms a basis for more functional strength. The more you can build isometric strength, the more your overall strength improves.

- **Improve body awareness.** This allows you to have better control over your body, to improve movement mechanics, to notice imbalances or inefficiencies, and to correct these.

- **Connect breath and movement.** This helps you notice and develop the connection between breathing and movement and to use this relationship to maximize physical performance.

- **Warm up well.** An additional use of isometric exercise is as a warm-up. Isometric exercises are great for improving muscle activation. They help to pump fresh blood into the target muscles, which prepares them for maximum efficiency during exercise. This helps to reduce strain on joints and makes for "smoother" movement during training.

For isometric and slower-moving exercise, build your practice with these workouts.	No-Impact Lower-Body Endurance (p. 54) · Hip Strength & Mobility (p. 58) · Knee Strength (p. 60) · Total Upper-Body Strength (p. 61) · Shoulder Strength (p. 62) · Full-Body Strength, Mobility & Injury Prevention (p. 72)

NO-IMPACT & LOW-IMPACT TRAINING

Most endurance training—especially running—is high-impact and very stressful on the joints. Yoga is entirely made up of low-impact and no-impact exercises, meaning there is minimal stress on your joints. Despite this, it's still a great way to build strength and endurance. So if you're not feeling up to a run, yoga is a great alternative to build endurance and strength without the "ouch" on your joints.

For low-impact exercise, build your practice with these workouts.	No-Impact Lower-Body Endurance (p. 54) · Ankle Stability (p. 57) · Hip Strength & Mobility (p. 58) · Knee Strength (p. 60) · Total Upper-Body Strength (p. 61) · Runner's Strength, Flexibility & Balance (p. 66) · Endurance Athlete's Strength, Mobility, Flexibility & Balance (p. 70)

FLEXIBILITY & MOBILITY TRAINING

Flexibility and mobility are critical to injury prevention as well as overall performance. You want your muscles to be flexible to avoid unnecessary strain on your joints, but you also want them to have mobility, which means strength combined with flexibility. Having more flexibility also allows your muscles to recover more quickly, decreasing your risk of injury from overtraining and allowing you to return to your workouts more adequately recovered. Mobility is important because this translates into improved performance and strength. However, flexibility is still the base of all mobility, so you'll need to continue to work on both. Mobility is particularly important to you as an endurance athlete because training usually involves movements that do not exercise the full range of motion of the joints. Exercises like lunges and squats—variations of which you'll find in any yoga workout—in which you are pushing your mobility levels are very important for joint stability, preventing injury, and addressing potentially dangerous muscle imbalances. Yoga, in particular, is very good for building this type of strength and mobility at your end range of motion to dramatically improve performance.

For mobility training, build your practice with these workouts.	Ankle Stability (p. 57) · Hip Strength & Mobility (p. 58) · Runner's Strength, Flexibility & Balance (p. 66) · Endurance Athlete's Strength, Mobility, Flexibility & Balance (p. 70) · Full-Body Strength, Mobility & Injury Prevention (p. 72) · Overall Hip Flexibility (p. 76) · Adductor & Hamstring Flexibility (p. 77) · Shoulder Flexibility (p. 80) · Foot & Ankle Mobility (p. 81) · Total Spine Mobility (p. 82) · Full-Body Flexibility & Mobility (p. 84)

BALANCE WORK

Balance is remaining steady, especially in compromised or unsteady positions, such as remaining stable in one-sided exercises or exercises where your weight is on one leg or standing on an unsteady surface. In the context of yoga, balance training generally refers to practicing stability while standing on one foot while executing a specific posture with your body. Balance is practical for you as an endurance athlete to help your body react to uneven terrain or unexpected obstacles. But the strength and mobility you build from practicing balance postures regularly is an extremely effective form of exercise for building muscle, as well. Balance work in particular helps to strengthen the ankles, knees, hips, and core. It also improves body awareness and helps you to notice imbalances between your left and right sides. The bottom line: balance work improves performance, builds strength, and lowers risk of injury.

For better balance, build your practice with these workouts.	Balance Strength (p. 53) · Balance for Hips, Ankles, Knees & Core (p. 56) · Ankle Stability (p. 57) · Hip Strength & Mobility (p. 58) · Knee Strength (p. 60)

RECOVERY TRAINING

Recovery training is helpful for any type of fitness, but perhaps even more so to endurance athletes because their training requires them to engage in such demanding, long-lasting workouts. Without recovery training, you're drastically lowering the training volume in which you can engage while maintaining a low risk of injury. Recovery training speeds up recovery. It lengthens muscles to relieve pressure on the joints. It helps to stimulate the parasympathetic nervous system, which switches the

body into recovery mode. For endurance athletes who are "in season," recovery training is especially important. As the mileage goes up, so too should your recovery work. Failure to do so increases risk of injury for overtraining, and you may find yourself sitting out for days or weeks if that happens. Yoga helps with this in three big ways:

1. The restorative stretches allow your muscles to relax, to release tension, to lengthen, and to recover.

2. The active recovery process of stretching (as opposed to sitting and doing nothing) also helps to flush dead tissue from broken down muscle fibers and speeds along recovery.

3. The slow, controlled breathing practiced while doing yoga helps to activate the body's parasympathetic nervous response, sending your body into a state of "rest and digest," encouraging your body to recover and replenish, as opposed to being stressed and ready to "fight or flight."

These benefits are *immediately* noticeable. Taking the time to practice yoga with an emphasis on recovery stretching and breathing allows you to return to your workouts feeling stronger and better rested. Your joints feel better and your movement feels smoother, and you're able to train more frequently and stick to your schedule.

For recovery training, build your practice with these workouts and poses.	**Workouts:** Knee Soreness Relief (p. 95) · Upper-Body & Shoulder Soreness Relief (p. 96) · Back Pain Relief (p. 98) · Total Spine Relief (p. 99) · Full-Body Restoration (p. 100) **Poses:** Bridge: Supported on Block (p. 111) · Child's Pose (p. 116) · Downdog: On Wall (p. 123) · Frog (p. 124) · Lizard (p. 134) · Pigeon (p. 138) · Reclined Strap Stretches (p. 142) · Standing Sidebend: On Wall (p. 159) · Thread the Needle (p. 160) · Triangle: Supported on Block (p. 165) · Wide-Legged Forward Fold (p. 170)

TRAINING ADVICE: Race Season vs Out of Season: If you don't already have an "off season" and an "on season", you should consider establishing one. During your off-season, you'll want to focus on building more strength and prepare for the stress of increased endurance training. During "in-season" training, focus more on endurance training and recovery workouts, and less on your strength-focused workouts.

PAIN POINTS

You probably have certain pain points, discomforts, or old injuries that force you to modify your training. A yoga practice does more than just help with recovery—it also strengthens the weaknesses that are at the root of these pain points. Yoga is also great for getting out in front of injuries before they happen, so you can use these workouts as prehab, too. Let's look at typical injuries, their causes, and the weaknesses that need to be addressed to fix them. Use the table to find the pain points that are keeping you from getting fitter. Find the corresponding workouts to begin improving.

AREA	SPECIFIC INJURY/ ISSUE	CAUSES	CORRECTIVE AREAS OF FOCUS	BUILD YOUR PRACTICE WITH THESE WORKOUTS AND POSES
FEET/ ANKLES	**Injuries:** Achilles tendinitis; Achilles tendon rupture; plantar fasciitis **Pains and discomforts:** Achilles tightness; calf strain; general feet pain	Lack of ankle strength Lack of ankle mobility Improper technique Flat feet or weak arches	Ankle mobility Ankle strength Arch strength Balance	**Workouts:** Balance Strength (p. 53) · Balance for Hips, Ankles, Knees & Core (p. 56) · Ankle Stability (p. 57) · Knee Strength (p. 60) · Resistance Athlete's Strength, Mobility, Flexibility & Balance (p. 68) · Foot & Ankle Mobility (p. 81) **Poses:** Airplane (p. 104) · Chair (p. 114) · Downdog (p. 122), High Lunge (p. 130) · Tree (p. 162) · Warrior 1 (p. 166) · Warrior 2 (p. 168) · Wide-Legged Forward Fold (p. 170)
KNEES	**Injuries:** Meniscus/ MCL tear; patellar tendinitis **Pains and discomforts:** General knee pain (a.k.a. runner's knee) during or after exercise	Lack of hip, ankle, and core stability and strength; lack of hip and ankle mobility; excessive high-impact training	Ankle mobility Ankle strength Balance Core strength General recovery stretching to prevent overtraining Hip mobility Hip strength	**Workouts:** Total Core Strength (p. 52) · Balance for Hips, Ankles, Knees & Core (p. 56) · Hip Strength & Mobility (p. 58) · Knee Strength (p. 60) · Muscular Imbalance Correction (p. 64) · Overall Hip Flexibility (p. 76) · Adductor & Hamstring Flexibility (p. 77) · Glute, Hip Flexor & Quadricep Flexibility (p. 78) · Foot & Ankle Mobility (p. 81) · Runner's Warm-Up (p. 91) · Knee Soreness Relief (p. 95) **Poses:** Airplane (p. 104) · Boat (p. 108) · Bridge (p. 110) · Chair (p. 114) · Cobra (p. 118) · Downdog (p. 122) · Frog (p. 124) · High Lunge (p. 130) · Horse (p. 132) · Lizard (p. 134) · Pigeon (p. 138) · Pyramid (p. 140) · Reclined Strap Stretches (p. 142) · Side Plank (p. 152) · Standing Bow (p. 156) · Tree (p. 162) · Triangle (p. 154) · Warrior 2 (p. 168)
LOWER BACK	**Injuries:** Herniated discs; slipped discs; spinal fusion surgery; degenerative discs; vertebral stress fractures **Pains and discomforts:** General, chronic, or exercise-induced lower-back pain	Lack of core and hip strength; lack of hip and spine mobility	Balance Core strength Hip mobility Hip strength Posture Spinal mobility	**Workouts:** Total Core Strength (p. 52) · Balance Strength (p. 53) · Hip Strength & Mobility (p. 58) · Knee Strength (p. 60) · Overall Hip Flexibility (p. 76) · Adductor & Hamstring Flexibility (p. 77) · Glute, Hip Flexor & Quadricep Flexibility (p. 78) · Total Spine Mobility (p. 82) · Back Pain Relief (p. 98) · Total Spine Relief (p. 30) **Poses:** Airplane (p. 104) · Boat (p. 108) · Bridge (p. 110) · Child's Pose (p. 116) · Chair (p. 114) · Cobra (p. 118) · Downdog (p. 122) · Frog (p. 124) Full Locust (p. 126) · Horse (p. 132) · Lizard (p. 134) · Pigeon (p. 138) · Reclined Strap Stretches (p. 142) · Reclined Twist (p. 144) Seated Twist (p. 148) · Side Plank (p. 152) · Standing Backbend (p. 154) · Standing Sidebend (p. 158) · Tree (p. 162)

AREA	SPECIFIC INJURY / ISSUE	CAUSES	CORRECTIVE AREAS OF FOCUS	BUILD YOUR PRACTICE WITH THESE WORKOUTS AND POSES
MIDDLE AND UPPER BACK	**Pains and discomforts:** Neck pain; middle- and upper-back pain	Lack of thoracic mobility; poor posture; upper-back weakness; core weakness	Core strength Posture Spinal mobility Spinal strength	**Workouts:** Total Core Strength (p. 52) · Balance Strength (p. 53) · Total Upper-Body Strength (p. 61) · Shoulder Strength (p. 62) · Muscular Imbalance Correction (p. 64) · Shoulder Flexibility (p. 80) · Total Spine Mobility (p. 82) · Warm-Up For Healthy Shoulders (p. 94) · Back Pain Relief (p. 98) · Total Spine Relief (p. 99) **Poses:** Boat (p. 108) · Bridge (p. 110) · Child's Pose (p. 116) · Cobra (p. 118) · Dolphin (p. 120) · Downdog (p. 122) · Full Locust (p. 126) · Reclined Twist (p. 144) · Seated Twist (p. 148) · Side Angle (p. 150) · Standing Backbend (p. 154) · Standing Bow (p. 156) · Standing Sidebend (p. 158) · Thread the Needle (p. 160) · Tree (p. 162) · Wide-Legged Forward Fold (p. 170)
HEAD AND NECK	**Pains and discomforts:** General neck pain	Lack of cervical mobility; poor posture; general neck weakness; lack of core strength	Core strength Hip mobility Hip strength Posture Spinal mobility Upper-back strength	**Workouts:** Balance for Hips, Ankles, Knees & Core (p. 56), Total Upper-Body Strength (p. 61) · Shoulder Strength (p. 62) · Muscular Imbalance Correction (p. 64) · Shoulder Flexibility (p. 80) · Total Spine Mobility (p. 82) · Full-Body Flexibility & Mobility (p. 84) · Warm-Up For Healthy Shoulders (p. 94) · Back Pain Relief (p. 98) · Total Spine Relief (p. 99) **Poses:** Boat (p. 108) · Child's Pose (p. 116) · Cobra (p. 118) · Dolphin (p. 120) · Downdog (p. 122) · Full Locust (p. 126) · Seated Twist (p. 148) · Side Angle (p. 150) · Standing Backbend (p. 154) · Standing Sidebend (p. 158) · Tree (p. 162) · Warrior 2 (p. 168)
SHOULDERS	**Injuries:** Rotator cuff tear; biceps tear; shoulder impingement **Pains and discomforts:** General shoulder pain	Lack of shoulder mobility and strength; poor posture	Shoulder mobility Upper-body strength	**Workouts:** Balance for Hips, Ankles, Knees & Core (p. 56), Total Upper-Body Strength (p. 61) · Shoulder Strength (p. 62) · Muscular Imbalance Correction (p. 64) · Shoulder Flexibility (p. 80) · Warm-Up For Healthy Shoulders (p. 94) · Upper-Body and Shoulder Soreness Relief (p. 96) **Poses:** Airplane: Warrior 3 (p. 104) · Boat (p. 108) · Child's Pose (p. 116) · Cobra (p. 118) · Dolphin (p. 120) · Downdog (p. 122) · Full Locust (p. 126) · High Lunge: Backbend and Twist (p. 131) · Side Angle (p. 150) · Side Plank (p. 152) · Standing Backbend (p. 154) · Standing Sidebend (p. 158) · Thread the Needle (p. 160) · Wide-Legged Forward Fold: With Strap and Twist (p. 171)

HOW TO PRACTICE YOGA WHEN YOU HAVE PAIN POINTS

While some yoga postures may be helpful, I do not recommend yoga as an alternative to physical therapy. To ensure you are doing the appropriate exercises to facilitate recovery, you should find a licensed physical therapist who focuses on exercise-based rehabilitation.

As a general rule of thumb: If it hurts, don't do it. While injured or recovering from injury, some of these postures will be accessible, while others will not. Discomfort is okay, but avoid sharp or shooting pain. Important Note: These guidelines are meant to address minor injuries, and they should not be used to replace the advice of a physical therapist or an orthopedic doctor. Every situation is unique, so make sure you have a proper conversation with a licensed medical professional before exercising with a significant injury.

For lower-body injuries: Avoid any weight-bearing or standing postures. This means that you should not do any exercises where you are placing weight on the affected leg. Focus on non-weight-bearing exercises instead.

For back injuries: Depending on the severity of the injury, generally you will want to stay active to facilitate recovery. Just make sure that the exercises are not causing you any pain. Keep range of motion limited; avoid deep forward folds, twists, or backbends.

For upper-body injuries: Many of the postures will be accessible, but you may have to modify how you use your hands. For example, if you have a shoulder injury, you're welcome to practice lunge-like yoga postures, but you should keep your arms relaxed at your sides instead of lifting them overhead.

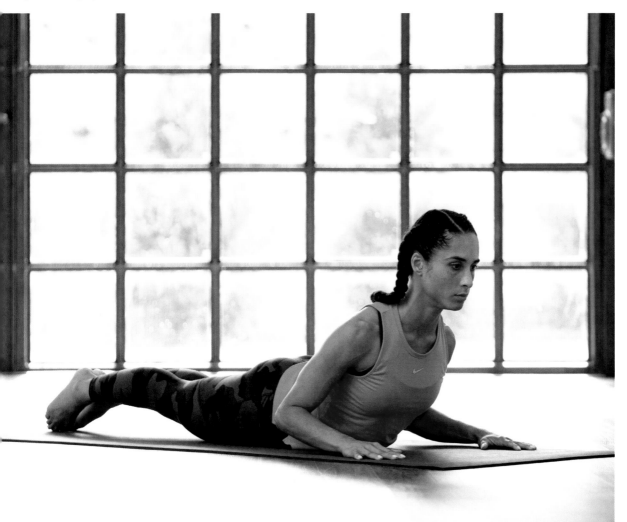

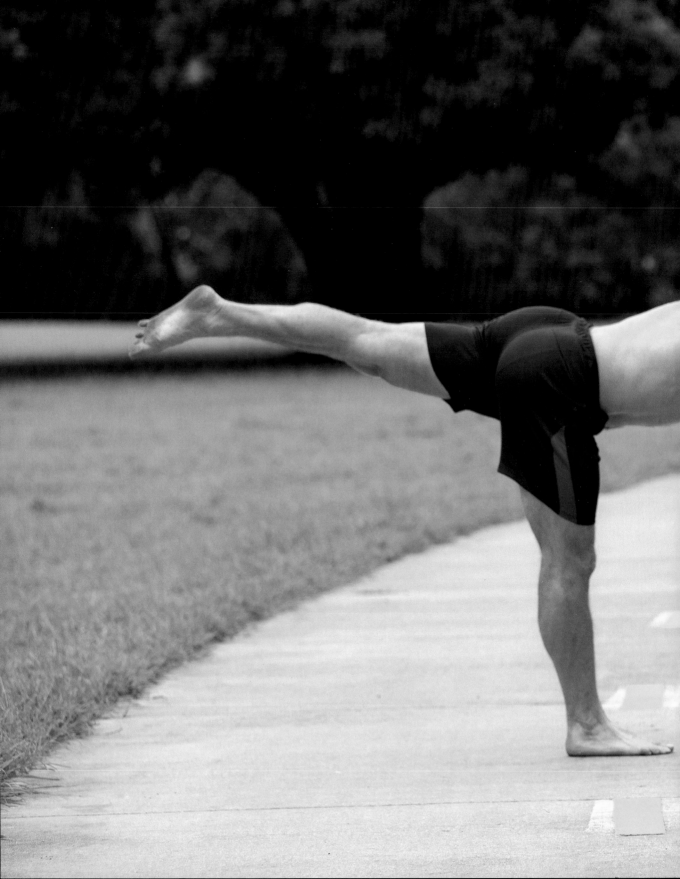

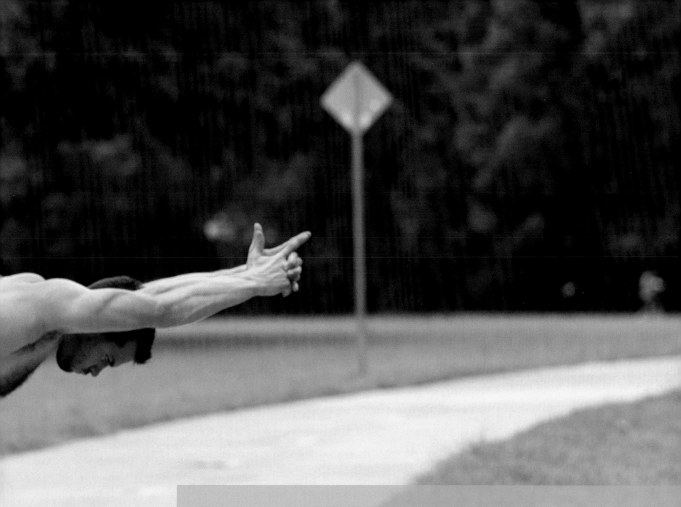

CHAPTER 4 »
TARGETED WORKOUTS

STRENGTH & INJURY-PREVENTION

These workouts are more intense routines that address a combination of strength, endurance, active mobility, and balance. They're meant to maximize muscle activation, challenge you on an individual level, and help you build strength in new ways. These workouts are great as standalone workouts, and many can also be used as warm-ups or finishers (a challenging ending to your workout).

TOTAL CORE STRENGTH

- Builds comprehensive core strength
- Strengthens hips, abs, and back
- Addresses root causes of lower-back and knee discomfort or pain

Total time: 11 minutes
Hold each posture for the recommended time.
No equipment required
Workout type: Warm-up, standalone

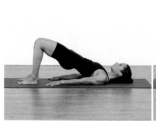

Bridge (p. 110)
» 60 seconds

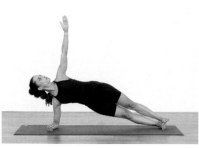

Bridge: Single-Leg (p. 111)
» 45 seconds per side

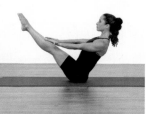

Boat (p. 108)
» 60 seconds

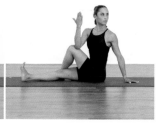

Seated Twist (p. 148)
» 45 seconds per side

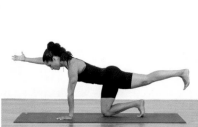

Side Plank (p. 152)
» 45 seconds per side

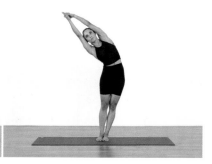

Bird Dog (p. 106)
» 30 seconds per side

Standing Sidebend (p. 158)
» 30 seconds per side

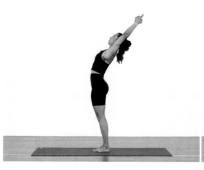

Standing Backbend (p. 154)
» 30 seconds

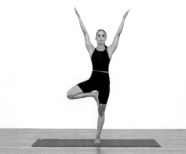

Tree (p. 162)
» 30 seconds per side

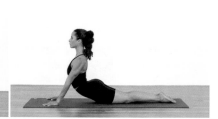

Cobra (p. 118)
» 45 seconds

BALANCE STRENGTH

- Builds strength in the muscles used during balancing: core, knees, hips, back, and ankles
- Reduces risk of injury in knees, ankles, and back

Total time: 9 minutes

Hold each posture for the recommended time.
No equipment required
Workout type: Warm-up, standalone

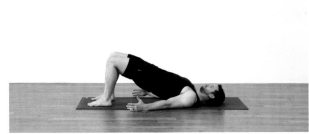

Bridge (p. 110)
» 60 seconds

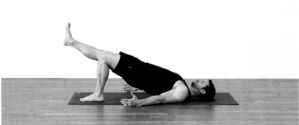

Bridge: Single-Leg (p. 111)
» 45 seconds per side

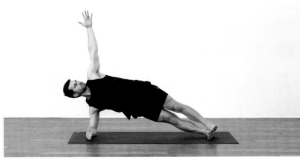

Side Plank (p. 152)
» 60 seconds per side

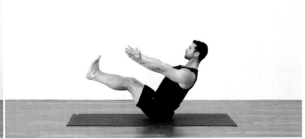

Boat (p. 108)
» 60 seconds

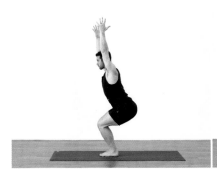

Chair (p. 114)
» 60 seconds

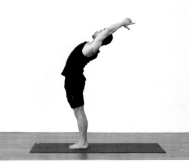

Standing Backbend (p. 154)
» 45 seconds

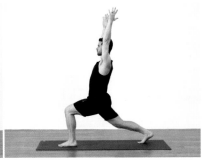

High Lunge (p. 130)
» 60 seconds per side

NO-IMPACT LOWER-BODY ENDURANCE

- Builds lower-body endurance with no-impact exercises
- Strengthens hips, core, back, and ankles

Total time: 9 minutes
Hold each posture for the recommended time.
No equipment required
Workout type: Standalone

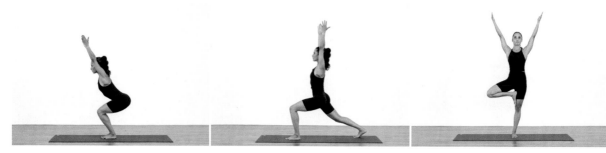

Chair (p. 114)
» 60 seconds

High Lunge (p. 130)
» 60 seconds per side

Tree (p. 162)
» 60 seconds per side

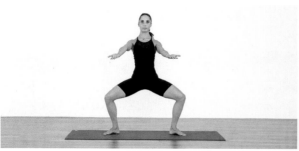

Horse (p. 132)
» 60 seconds

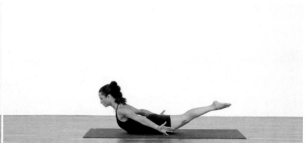

Full Locust (p. 126)
» 30 seconds

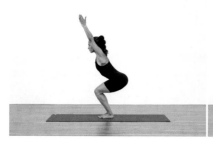

Chair (p. 114)
» 30 seconds

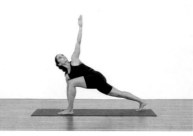

Runner's Lunge Twist (p. 146)
» 30 seconds per side

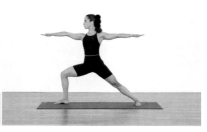

Warrior 2 (p. 168)
» 30 seconds per side

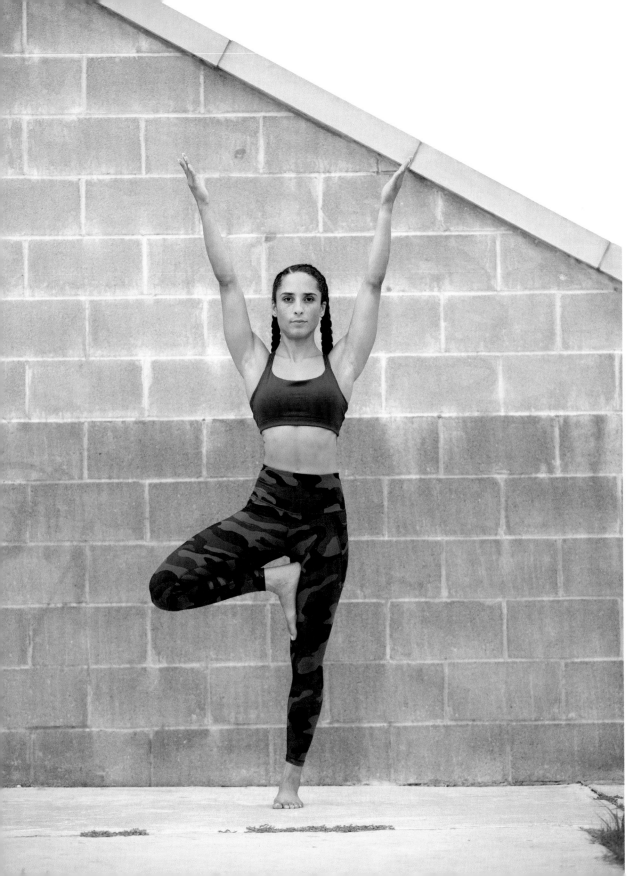

BALANCE FOR HIPS, ANKLES, KNEES & CORE

- Improves full-body balance
- Strengthens core, hips, and ankles
- Reduces risk of injury in knees, ankles, and back

Total time: 9 minutes

Hold each posture for the recommended time.
No equipment required
Workout type: Warm-up, standalone

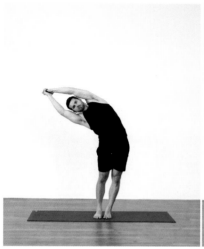

Standing Sidebend (p. 158)
» 45 seconds per side

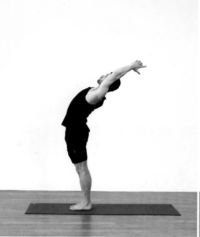

Standing Backbend (p. 154)
» 45 seconds

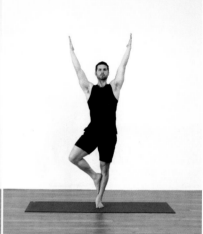

Tree (p. 162)
» 60 seconds per side

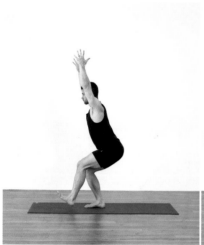

Chair: Single-Leg (p. 115)
» 30 seconds per side

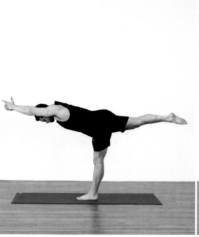

Airplane or Warrior 3 (p. 104)
» 60 seconds per side

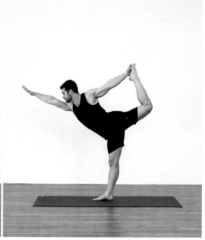

Standing Bow (p. 156)
» 60 seconds per side

ANKLE STABILITY

- Builds ankle stability
- Improves balance
- Strengthens knees and ankles

Total time: 10 minutes
Hold each posture for the recommended time.
Equipment: Blocks (optional)
Workout type: Standalone

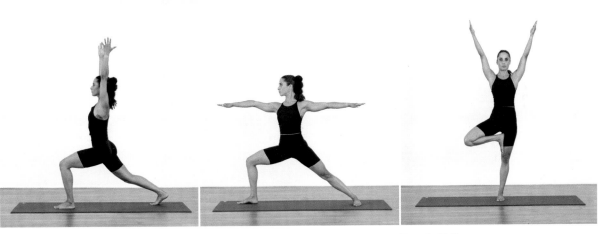

High Lunge (p. 130)
» 60 seconds per side

Warrior 2 (p. 168)
» 60 seconds per side

Tree (p. 162)
» 60 seconds per side

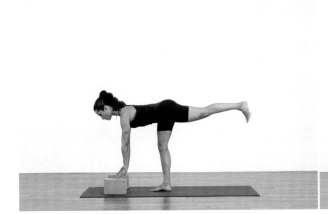

Airplane (Supported on Blocks; optional) (p. 104)
» 60 seconds per side

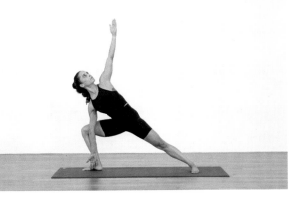

Side Angle (p. 150)
» 60 seconds per side

HIP STRENGTH & MOBILITY

- Increases functional strength and mobility in hips
- Builds core strength
- Reduces load on knees and lower back

Total time: 10 minutes
Hold each posture for the recommended time.
No equipment required
Workout type: Warm-up, standalone

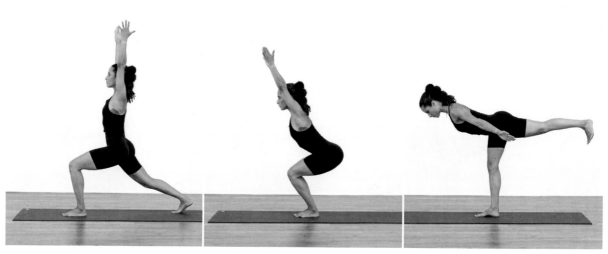

High Lunge (p. 130)
» 60 seconds per side

Chair (p. 114)
» 60 seconds

Airplane (p. 104)
» 60 seconds per side

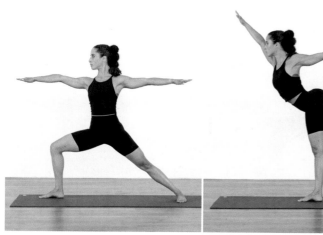

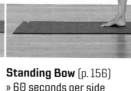

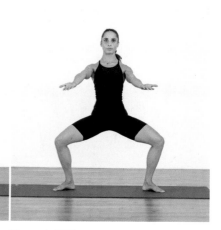

Warrior 2 (p. 168)
» 60 seconds per side

Standing Bow (p. 156)
» 60 seconds per side

Horse (p. 132)
» 60 seconds

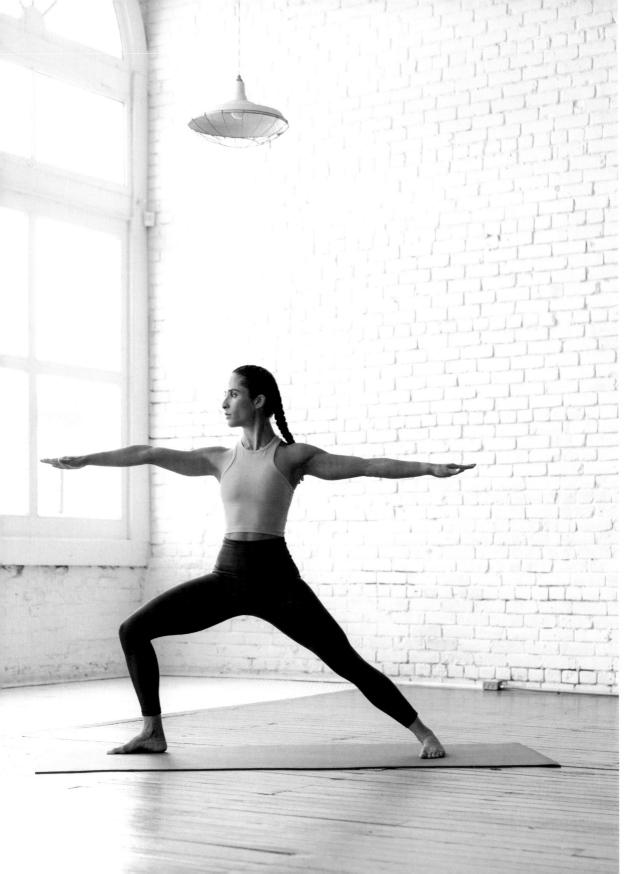

KNEE STRENGTH

- Comprehensively addresses knee strength and stability
- Reduces strain on knees by strengthening supporting areas—hips, core, and ankles
- Increases mobility, balance, and endurance

Total time: 11 minutes

Hold each posture for the recommended time.
No equipment required
Workout type: Warm-up, standalone

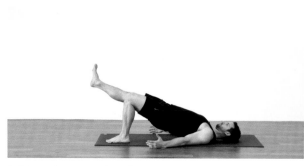

Bridge: Single-Leg (p. 111)
» 60 seconds per side

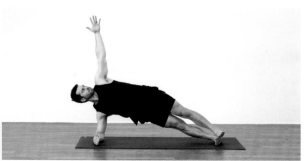

Side Plank (p. 152)
» 60 seconds per side

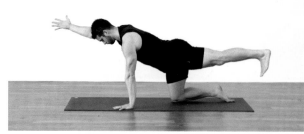

Bird Dog (p. 106)
» 30 seconds per side

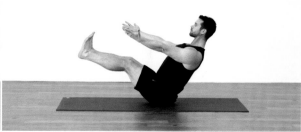

Boat (p. 108)
» 30 seconds

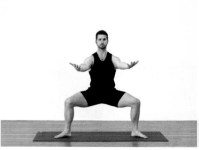

Horse (p. 132)
» 60 seconds

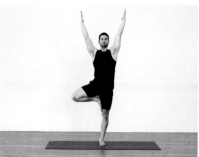

Tree (p. 162)
» 60 seconds per side

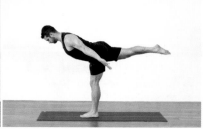

Airplane (p. 104)
» 60 seconds per side

TOTAL UPPER-BODY STRENGTH

- Builds strength, endurance, and mobility in shoulders, chest, and upper back
- Increases overall core strength
- Opens chest and helps to realign proper posture

Total time: 10 minutes
Hold each posture for the recommended time.
No equipment required
Workout type: Standalone

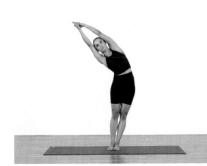

Standing Sidebend (p. 158)
» 60 seconds per side

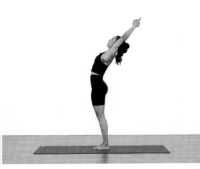

Standing Backbend (p. 154)
» 60 seconds

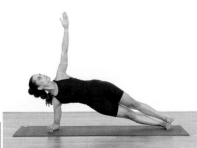

Side Plank (p. 152)
» 60 seconds per side

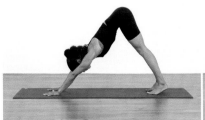

Downdog (p. 122)
» 60 seconds

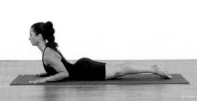

Cobra (p. 118)
» 60 seconds

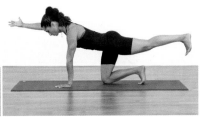

Bird Dog (p. 106)
» 30 seconds per side

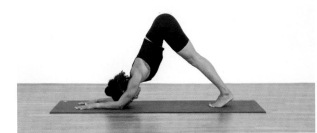

Dolphin (p. 120)
» 60 seconds

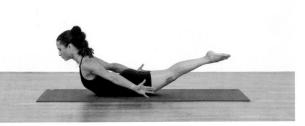

Full Locust (p. 126)
» 60 seconds

SHOULDER STRENGTH

- Improves upper-body strength
- Increases shoulder mobility and helps prevent shoulder injury
- Improves breathing patterns
- Reduces strain in back and neck

Total time: 10 minutes
Hold each posture for the recommended time.
Equipment: Strap
Workout type: Warm-up, standalone

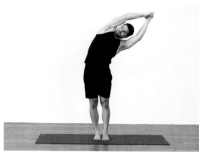

Standing Sidebend (p. 158)
» 45 seconds per side

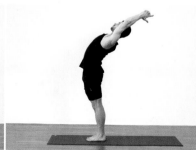

Standing Backbend (p. 154)
» 30 seconds

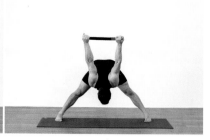

**Wide-Legged Forward Fold:
With Strap** (p. 170)
» 60 seconds

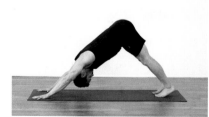

Downdog (p. 122)
» 60 seconds

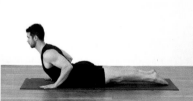

Cobra (p. 118)
» 45 seconds

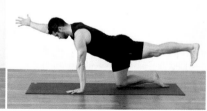

Bird Dog (p. 106)
» 45 seconds per side

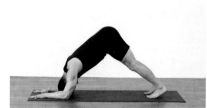

Dolphin (p. 120)
» 60 seconds

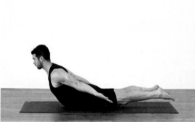

Full Locust (p. 126)
» 45 seconds

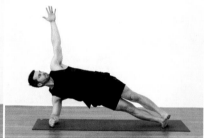

Side Plank (p. 152)
» 60 seconds per side

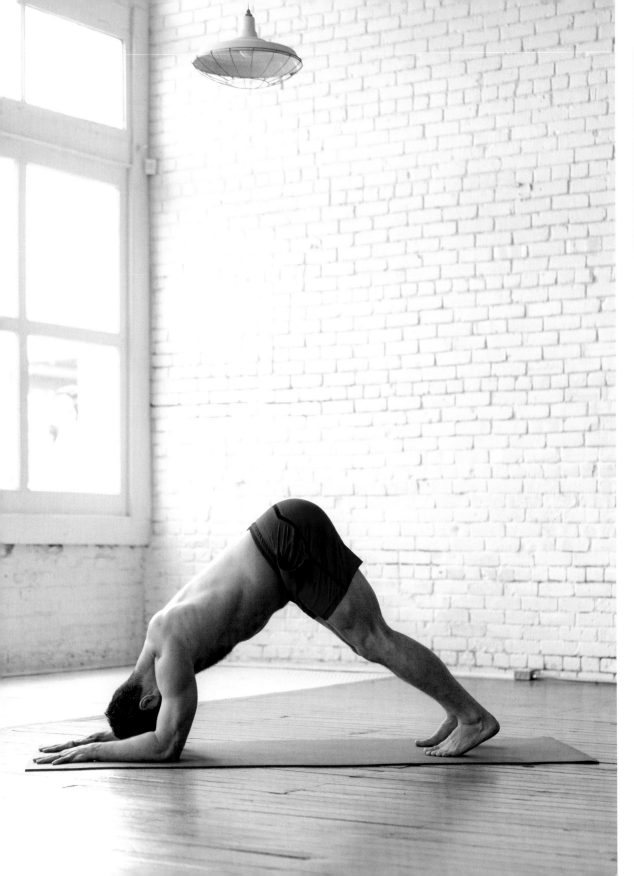

MUSCULAR IMBALANCE CORRECTION

- Builds strength and increases mobility in hips, core, back, and shoulders
- Reduces risk of injury for those who sit or are inactive for longer periods
- Improves posture for office workers (and perfect for the weekend warrior!)

Total time: 11 minutes
Hold each posture for the recommended time.
Equipment: Strap
Workout type: Standalone, warm-up

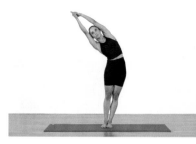

Standing Sidebend (p. 158)
» 60 seconds per side

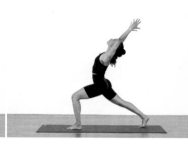

High Lunge: Backbend (p. 131)
» 60 seconds per side

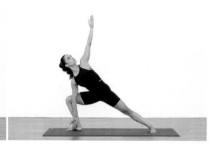

Side Angle (p. 150)
» 60 seconds per side

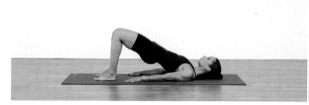

Bridge (p. 110)
» 60 seconds

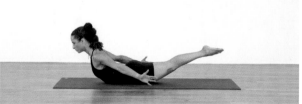

Full Locust (p. 126)
» 60 seconds

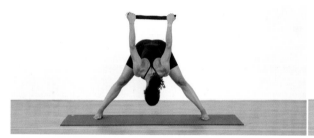

Wide-Legged Forward Fold: With Strap (p. 171)
» 60 seconds

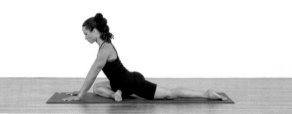

Pigeon (p. 138)
» 60 seconds per side

TRANSVERSE & FRONTAL PLANE MOVEMENTS

- Comprehensively strengthens core, especially for the endurance athlete
- Improves twisting and rotation for frontal plane (side-to-side) movements

Total time: 10 Minutes

Hold each posture for the recommended time.

No equipment required

Workout type: Warm-up, standalone

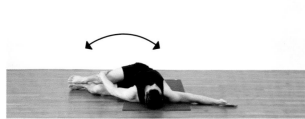

Reclined Twist, plus Reps (p. 144)
» 45 seconds per side, then 5 reps per side

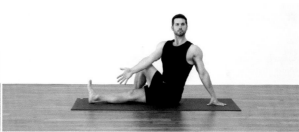

Seated Twist (p. 148)
» 30 seconds per side

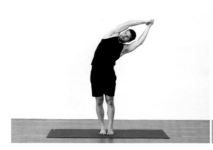

Standing Sidebend (p. 158)
» 45 seconds per side

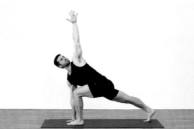

Runner's Lunge Twist (p. 146)
» 30 seconds per side

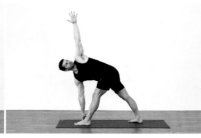

Triangle: Revolved (p. 165)
» 45 seconds per side

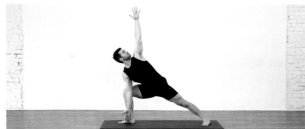

Side Angle (p. 150)
» 45 seconds per side

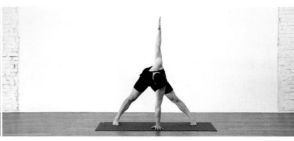

Wide-Legged Forward Fold: Twist (p. 170)
» 30 seconds per side

RUNNER'S STRENGTH, FLEXIBILITY & BALANCE

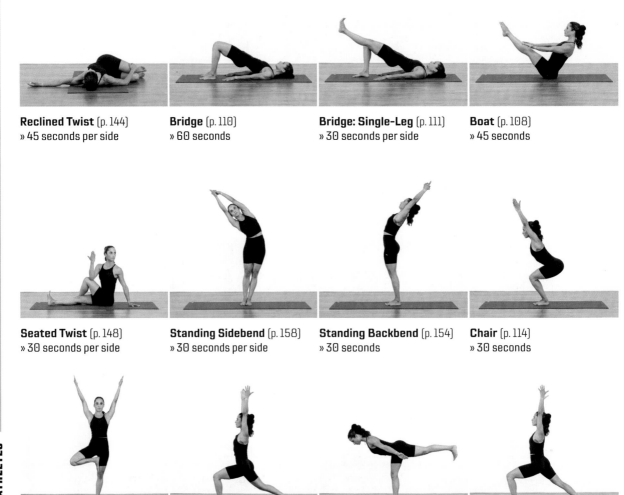

Reclined Twist (p. 144)
» 45 seconds per side

Bridge (p. 110)
» 60 seconds

Bridge: Single-Leg (p. 111)
» 30 seconds per side

Boat (p. 108)
» 45 seconds

Seated Twist (p. 148)
» 30 seconds per side

Standing Sidebend (p. 158)
» 30 seconds per side

Standing Backbend (p. 154)
» 30 seconds

Chair (p. 114)
» 30 seconds

Tree (p. 162)
» 45 seconds per side

High Lunge (p. 130)
» 45 seconds per side

Airplane (p. 104)
» 45 seconds per side

Warrior 1 (p. 166)
» 45 seconds per side

- Full-body, full-length workout that addresses common weaknesses, movement gaps, and imbalances in runners
- Strengthens and improves mobility in lower body and back
- Reduces strain on joints during exercise; a great no-impact alternative to an endurance workout

Total time: 30 minutes
Hold each posture for the recommended time.
Equipment: Strap
Workout type: Standalone

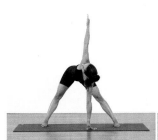

Wide-Legged Forward Fold: Twist (p. 171)
» 30 seconds per side

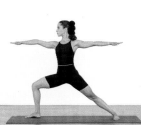

Warrior 2 (p. 168)
» 45 seconds per side

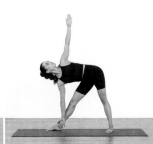

Triangle (p. 164)
» 45 seconds per side

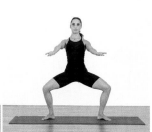

Horse (p. 132)
» 60 seconds

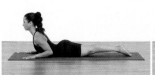

Cobra (p. 118)
» 30 seconds

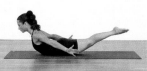

Full Locust (p. 126)
» 30 seconds

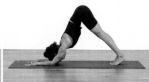

Dolphin (p. 120)
» 30 seconds

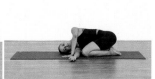

Thread the Needle (p. 160)
» 45 seconds per side

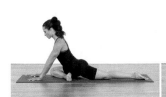

Pigeon (p. 138)
» 60 seconds per side

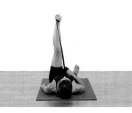

Hamstring Strap Stretch (p. 142)
» 60 seconds per side

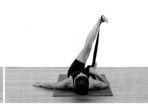

Abductor Strap Stretch (p. 143)
» 60 seconds per side

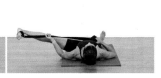

Adductor Strap Stretch (p. 143)
» 60 seconds per side

RESISTANCE ATHLETE'S STRENGTH, MOBILITY, FLEXIBILITY & BALANCE

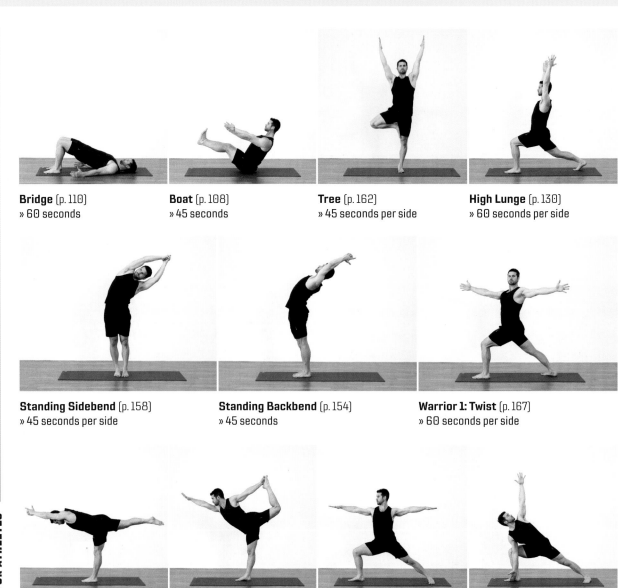

Bridge (p. 110)
» 60 seconds

Boat (p. 108)
» 45 seconds

Tree (p. 162)
» 45 seconds per side

High Lunge (p. 130)
» 60 seconds per side

Standing Sidebend (p. 158)
» 45 seconds per side

Standing Backbend (p. 154)
» 45 seconds

Warrior 1: Twist (p. 167)
» 60 seconds per side

Warrior 3 (p. 105)
» 45 seconds per side

Standing Bow (p. 156)
» 45 seconds per side

Warrior 2 (p. 168)
» 45 seconds per side

Side Angle (p. 150)
» 30 seconds per side

- Full-body, full-length workout that addresses common weaknesses and training gaps in weight training
- Combination of intense strength, mobility, and balance work, as well as less-intense flexibility work
- Great for non-training days

Total time: 27 minutes

Hold each posture for the recommended time.
No equipment required
Workout type: Standalone

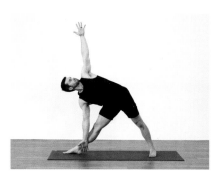

Triangle (p. 164)
» 30 seconds per side

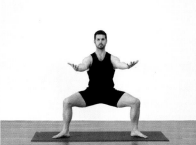

Horse (p. 132)
» 60 seconds per side

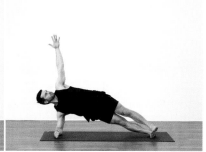

Side Plank (p. 152)
» 45 seconds per side

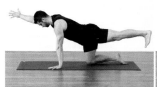

Bird Dog (p. 106)
» 30 seconds per side

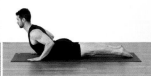

Cobra (p. 118)
» 30 seconds

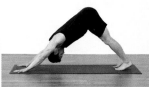

Downdog (p. 122)
» 60 seconds

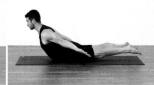

Full Locust (p. 126)
» 30 seconds

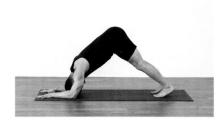

Dolphin (p. 120)
» 45 seconds

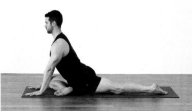

Pigeon (p. 138)
» 60 seconds per side

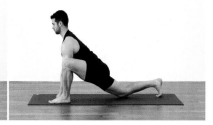

Lizard (p. 134)
» 60 seconds per side

ENDURANCE ATHLETE'S STRENGTH, MOBILITY, FLEXIBILITY & BALANCE

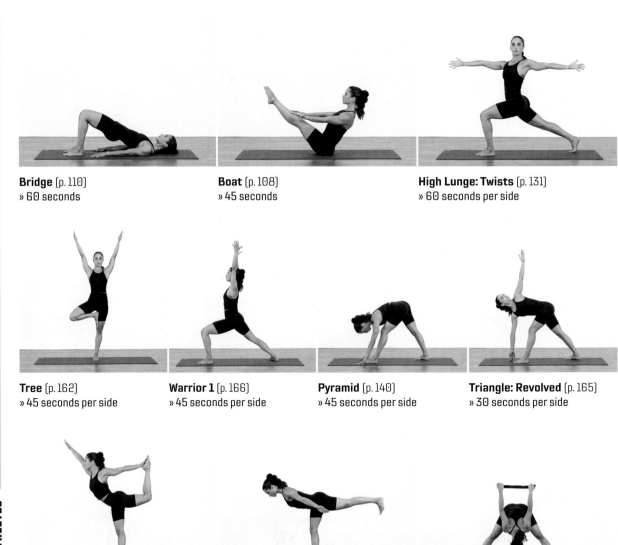

Bridge (p. 110)
» 60 seconds

Boat (p. 108)
» 45 seconds

High Lunge: Twists (p. 131)
» 60 seconds per side

Tree (p. 162)
» 45 seconds per side

Warrior 1 (p. 166)
» 45 seconds per side

Pyramid (p. 140)
» 45 seconds per side

Triangle: Revolved (p. 165)
» 30 seconds per side

Standing Bow (p. 156)
» 45 seconds per side

Airplane (p. 104)
» 45 seconds per side

Wide-Legged Forward Fold: With Strap (p. 171)
» 60 seconds

- Full-body, full-length workout that addresses common weaknesses and training gaps of endurance athletes
- Combination of intense strength, mobility, and balance and less-intense flexibility work
- Great for non-training days

Total time: 26 minutes
Hold each posture for the recommended time.
Equipment: Strap
Workout type: Standalone

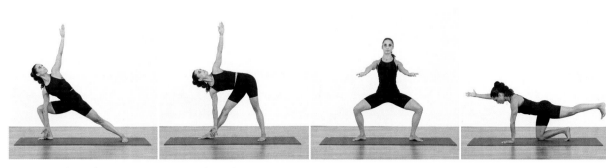

Side Angle (p. 150)
» 45 seconds per side

Triangle (p. 164)
» 30 seconds per side

Horse (p. 132)
» 60 seconds

Bird Dog (p. 106)
» 45 seconds per side

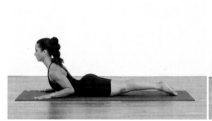

Cobra (p. 118)
» 30 seconds

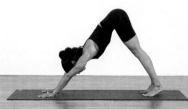

Downdog (p. 122)
» 60 seconds

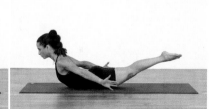

Full Locust (p. 126)
» 30 seconds

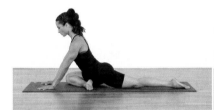

Pigeon (p. 138)
» 60 seconds per side

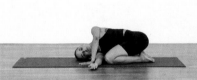

Thread the Needle (p. 160)
» 45 seconds per side

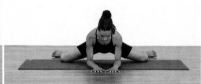

Frog (p. 124)
» 2 minutes

FULL-BODY STRENGTH, MOBILITY & INJURY-PREVENTION

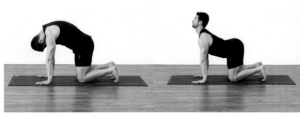

Cat-Cow (p. 112)
» 5–10 reps

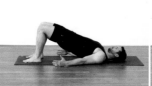

Bridge (p. 110)
» 60 seconds

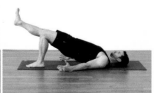

Bridge: Single-Leg (p. 111)
» 30 seconds per side

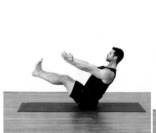

Boat (p. 108)
» 45 seconds

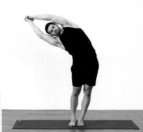

Standing Sidebend (p. 158)
» 45 seconds per side

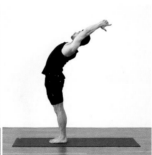

Standing Backbend (p. 154)
» 45 seconds

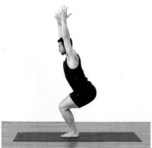

Chair (p. 114)
» 30 seconds

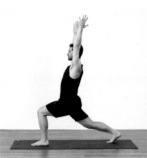

High Lunge (p. 130)
» 60 seconds per side

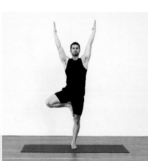

Tree (p. 162)
» 60 seconds per side

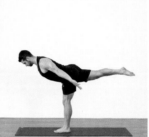

Airplane (p. 104)
» 45 seconds per side

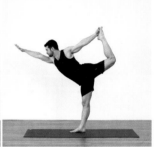

Standing Bow (p. 156)
» 45 seconds per side

- Full-body, full-length workout that builds comprehensive strength and mobility
- Increases active range of motion
- Improves core strength, balance, and muscle activation

Total time: 24 minutes
Hold each posture for the recommended time.
Equipment: Strap
Workout type: Standalone

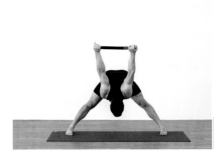

Wide-Legged Forward Fold: With Strap (p. 171)
» 60 seconds

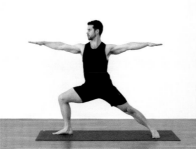

Warrior 2 (p. 168)
» 45 seconds per side

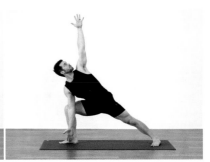

Side Angle (p. 150)
» 45 seconds per side

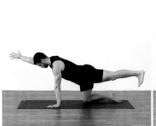

Bird Dog (p. 106)
» 45 seconds per side

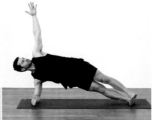

Side Plank (p. 152)
» 45 seconds per side

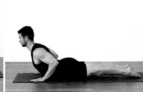

Cobra (p. 118)
» 30 seconds

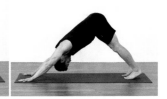

Downdog (p. 122)
» 60 seconds

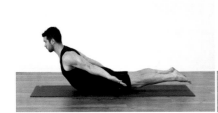

Full Locust (p. 126)
» 30 seconds

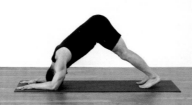

Dolphin (p. 120)
» 45 seconds

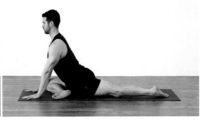

Pigeon (p. 138)
» 60 seconds per side

FLEXIBILITY

These workouts focus on increasing overall range of motion, including both passive and active mobility. Routines may use a combination of intense mobility- and strength-focused postures, as well as less-intense flexibility- and stretching-focused postures. Emphasis here is placed on using breathing to calm the nervous system and allow your muscles to relax and stretch, so as to maximize the benefits of your time and effort spent working on flexibility. Avoid gritting your teeth or tensing your shoulders and face, and concentrate on relaxing into the stretches.

OVERALL HIP FLEXIBILITY

- Builds flexibility in all major muscle groups of the hips, including hamstrings, glutes, adductors, abductors, and quadriceps
- Reduces strain on knees and back

Total time: 10 minutes

Hold each posture for the recommended time.

Equipment: Strap

Workout type: Standalone, recovery

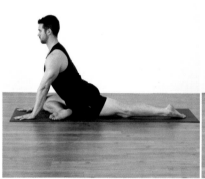

Pigeon (p. 138)
» 75 seconds per side

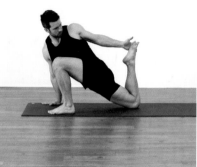

Lizard: Reachback (p. 135)
» 75 seconds per side

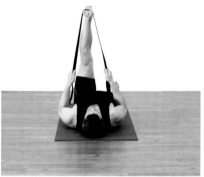

Hamstring Strap Stretch (p. 142)
» 45 seconds per side

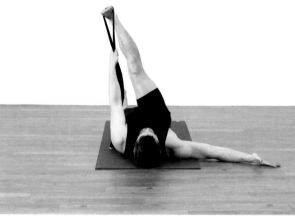

Abductor Strap Stretch (p. 143)
» 45 seconds per side

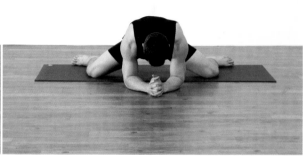

Frog (p. 124)
» 2 minutes

ADDUCTOR & HAMSTRING FLEXIBILITY

- Increases overall range of motion of adductors and hamstrings
- Reduces strain on back and knees
- Lowers risk of soft-tissue injury in hips, back, and knees

Total time: 11 minutes

Hold each posture for the recommended time.

Equipment: Block, strap

Workout type: Standalone, cooldown

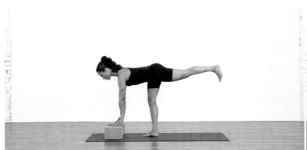

Airplane: Supported on Blocks (p. 105)
» 60 seconds per side

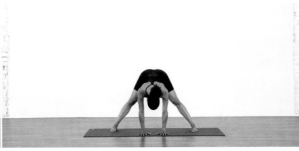

Wide-Legged Forward Fold (p. 170)
» 60 seconds

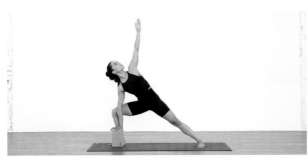

Side Angle: Supported on Block (p. 151)
» 60 seconds per side

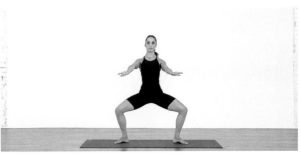

Horse (p. 132)
» 60 seconds

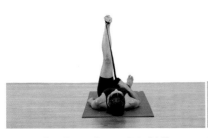

Hamstring Strap Stretch (p. 142)
» 60 seconds per side

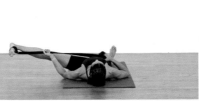

Adductor Strap Stretch (p. 143)
» 60 seconds per side

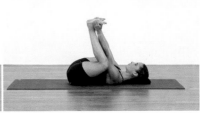

Happy Baby (p. 128)
» 60 seconds

GLUTE, HIP FLEXOR & QUADRICEP FLEXIBILITY

- Increases overall range of motion in glutes, hip flexors, and quadriceps
- Reduces strain on back and knees
- Lowers risk of soft-tissue injury in hips and knees

Total time: 10 minutes

Hold each posture for the recommended time.

Equipment: Strap

Workout type: Cooldown, standalone

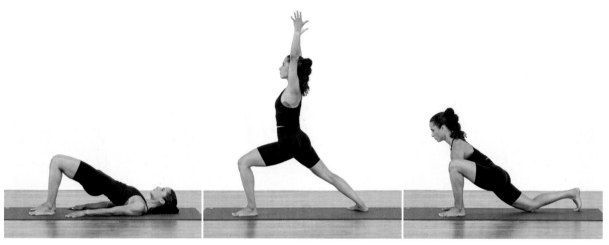

Bridge (p. 110)
» 60 seconds

Warrior 1 (p. 166)
» 60 seconds per side

Lizard (p. 134)
» 60 seconds per side

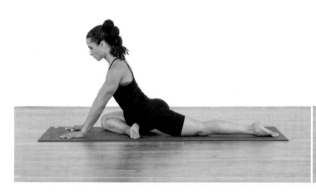

Pigeon (p. 138)
» 60 seconds per side

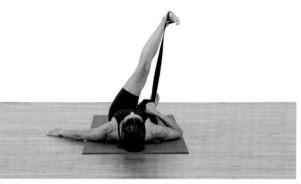

Abductor Strap Stretch (p. 143)
» 90 seconds per side

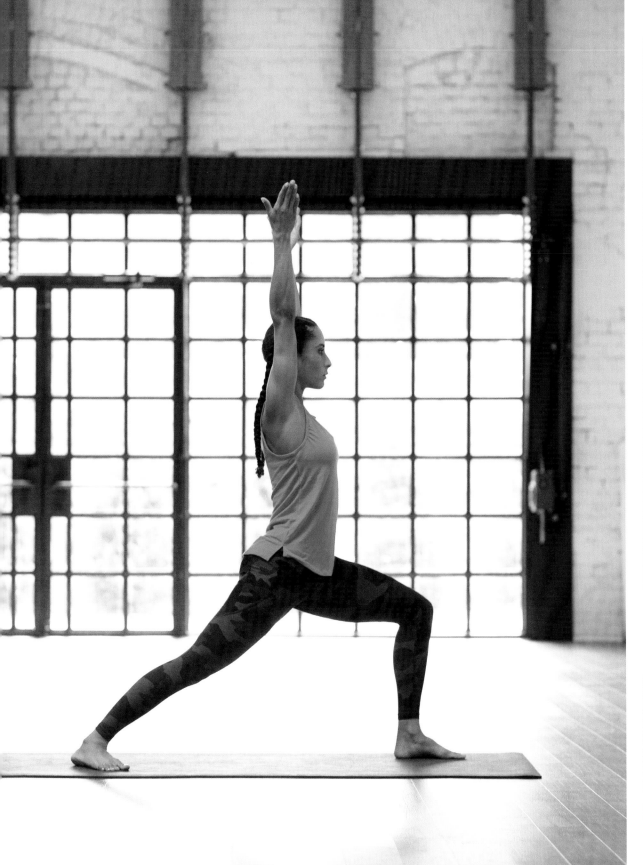

SHOULDER FLEXIBILITY

- Increases overall shoulder and upper-back flexibility
- Builds strength in upper back
- Corrects common muscular imbalances in upper body

Total time: 10 minutes
Hold each posture for the recommended time.
Equipment: Blocks, strap
Workout type: Standalone

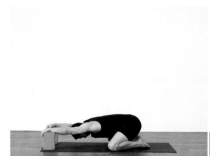

Child's Pose: Supported on Blocks
(p. 117)
» 90 seconds

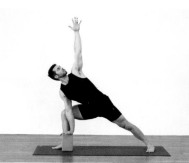

Side Angle: Supported on Block
(p. 151)
» 45 seconds per side

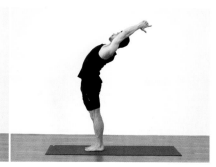

Standing Backbend (p. 154)
» 60 seconds

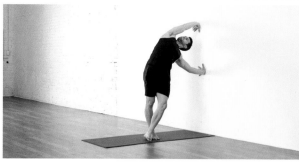

Standing Sidebend (On Wall; optional) (p. 158)
» 45 seconds per side

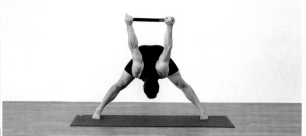

Wide-legged Forward Fold: With Strap (p. 171)
» 60 seconds

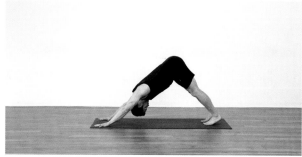

Downdog (On Wall; optional) (p. 122)
» 90 seconds

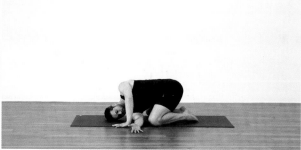

Thread the Needle (p. 160)
» 60 seconds per side

FOOT & ANKLE MOBILITY

- Helps resolve plantar fasciitis or Achilles tendinitis
- Increases strength and mobility in the feet, ankles, and hips
- Reduces strain on knees and lower back

Total time: 10 minutes

Hold each posture for the recommended time.

Equipment: Blocks, strap

Workout type: Standalone

Warrior 1 (p. 166)
» 60 seconds per side

Tree (p. 162)
» 45 seconds per side

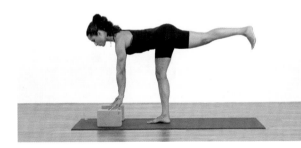

Airplane: Supported on Blocks (p. 105)
» 45 seconds per side

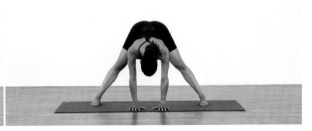

Wide-Legged Forward Fold (p. 170)
» 90 seconds

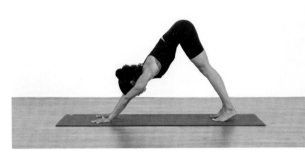

Downdog (On Wall; optional) (p. 122)
» 90 seconds

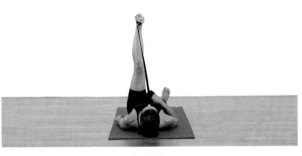

Hamstring Strap Stretch (p. 142)
» 60 seconds per side

TOTAL SPINE MOBILITY

- Increases mobility in all areas of the spine
- Reduces overall stiffness in back and improves movement fluidity
- Builds functional range of motion in spine

Total time: 11 minutes

Hold each posture for the recommended time.

No equipment required

Workout type: Warm-up, standalone

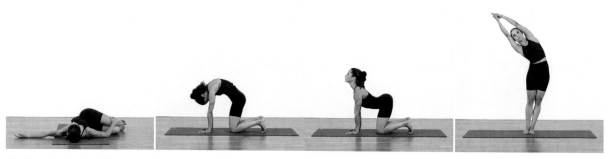

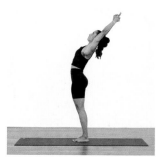

Reclined Twist (p. 144)
» 45 seconds per side

Cat-Cow (p. 112)
» 5–10 reps

Standing Sidebend (p. 158)
» 45 seconds per side

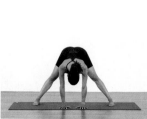
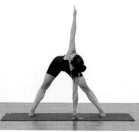
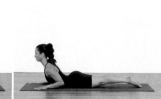

Standing Backbend (p. 154)
» 45 seconds

Wide-Legged Forward Fold (p. 170)
» 45 seconds

Wide-Legged Forward Fold: With Twist (p. 171)
» 30 seconds per side

Cobra (p. 118)
» 45 seconds

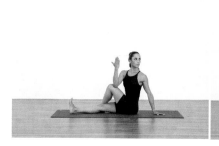
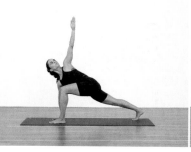
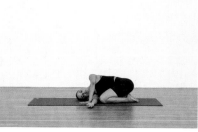

Seated Twist (p. 148)
» 45 seconds per side

Runner's Lunge Twist (p. 146)
» 30 seconds per side

Thread the Needle (p. 160)
» 45 seconds per side

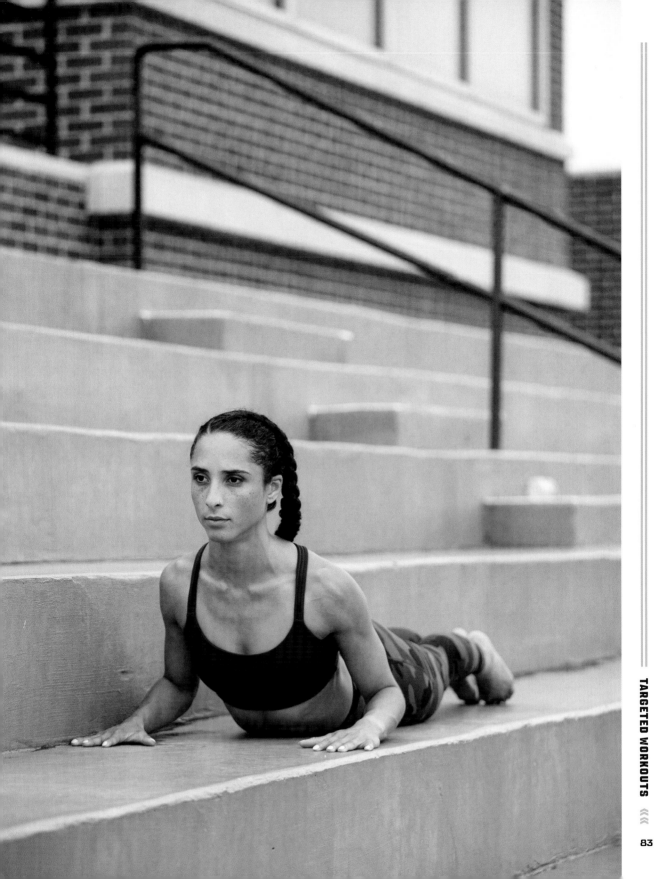

FULL-BODY FLEXIBILITY & MOBILITY

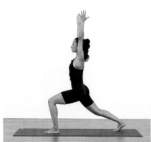

High Lunge (p. 130)
» 45 seconds per side

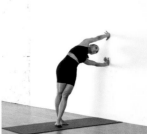

Standing Sidebend: On Wall (p. 159)
» 45 seconds per side

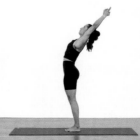

Standing Backbend (p. 154)
» 45 seconds

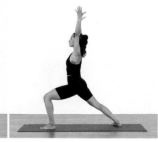

Warrior 1 (p. 166)
» 60 seconds per side

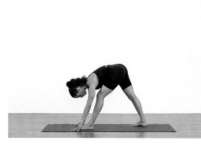

Pyramid (p. 140)
» 45 seconds per side

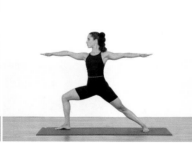

Warrior 2 (p. 168)
» 30 seconds per side

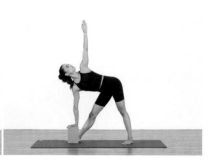

Triangle (Supported on Block; optional) (p. 164)
» 45 seconds per side

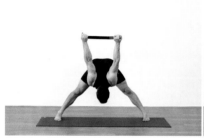

Wide-legged Forward Fold: With Strap (p. 171)
» 60 seconds

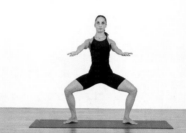

Horse (p. 132)
» 60 seconds

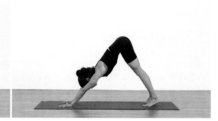

Downdog (p. 122)
» 60 seconds

- Full-body, full-length workout that increases overall range of motion
- Reduces muscle tightness to relieve joint discomfort
- Relieves stress and promotes recovery
- Starts with active, mobility-focused postures and ends with more passive, flexibility-focused stretches

Total time: 29 minutes
Hold each posture for the recommended time.
Equipment: Block (optional), strap
Workout type: Standalone

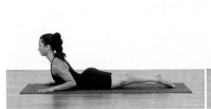

Cobra (p. 118)
» 30 seconds

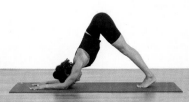

Dolphin (p. 120)
» 45 seconds

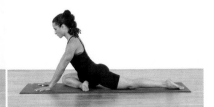

Pigeon (p. 138)
» 90 seconds per side

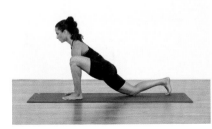

Lizard (p. 134)
» 60 seconds per side

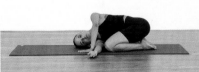

Thread the Needle (p. 160)
» 45 seconds per side

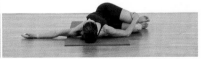

Reclined Twist (p. 144)
» 45 seconds per side

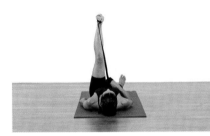

Hamstring Strap Stretch (p. 142)
» 60 seconds per side

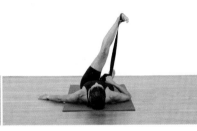

Abductor Strap Stretch (p. 143)
» 60 seconds per side

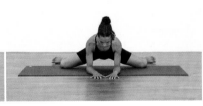

Frog (p. 124)
» 2 minutes

WARM-UPS, COOLDOWNS & RESTORATIVE WORKOUTS

Warm-up routines are designed to be used as a warm-up for another workout. These routines focus on activating key muscles used during exercise to reduce strain on joints, improve fluidity of motion, and decrease your risk of injury. Postures are generally held for a shorter duration, and the emphasis is on strength and mobility. Passive stretching is avoided.

Cooldown and restorative workouts are relaxed routines focused on passive flexibility and stretching. The goal of these restorative routines is to help release tension from your muscles, relieve stiffness or aching in your joints, and relax the central nervous system. Emphasis should be placed on long, relaxed breathing in combination with longer-held stretches. Ensure your face, shoulders, and neck are relaxed. Start stretches at a level 3 or 4 out of 10 with respect to intensity, and then breathe deeper into the stretch with each successive exhale. Use these immediately after a workout, the evening of, or even the day after.

ALL-PURPOSE WARM-UP TO PREVENT JOINT PAIN DURING WORKOUTS

- Prepares body for pain-free exercise or workout
- Builds muscle activation in key core, hip, shoulder, and ankle muscles

Total time: 5 minutes

Hold each posture for the recommended time.

No equipment required

Workout type: Warm-up, standalone

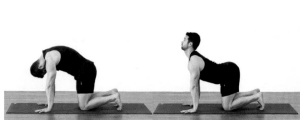

Cat-Cow (p. 112)
» 5–10 reps

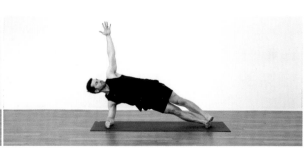

Cobra (p. 118)
» 30 seconds

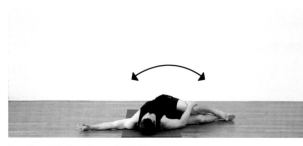

Reclined Twist: Reps (p. 145)
» 5 reps per side

Side Plank (p. 152)
» 30 seconds per side

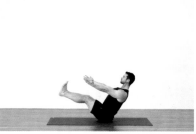

Boat (p. 108)
» 30 seconds

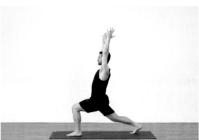

High Lunge (p. 130)
» 30 seconds per side

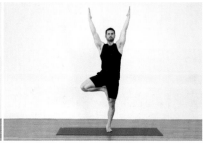

Tree (p. 162)
» 30 seconds per side

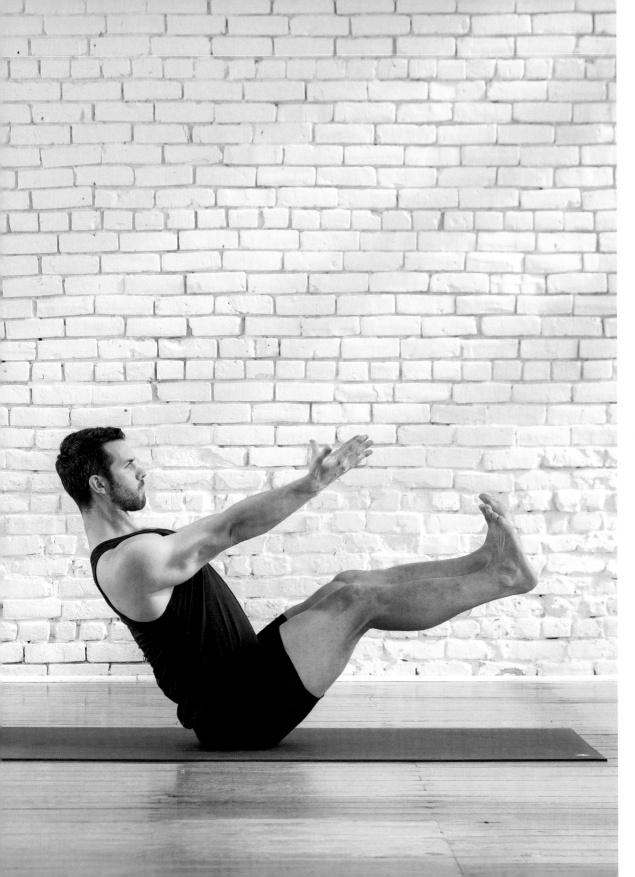

ENDURANCE ATHLETE'S WARM-UP

- Activates key muscles involved in endurance sports, such as running, cycling, and swimming
- Prepares joints for healthy, pain-free movement
- Reduces stiffness in back, knees, and shoulders

Total time: 7 minutes

Hold each posture for the recommended time.

No equipment required

Workout type: Warm-up, standalone

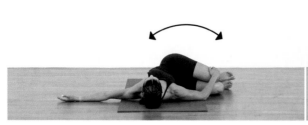

Reclined Twist: Reps (p. 145)
» 5 reps per side

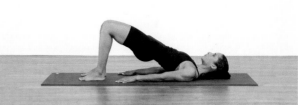

Bridge (p. 110)
» 60 seconds

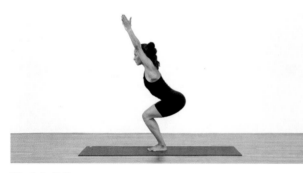

Chair (p. 114)
» 30 seconds

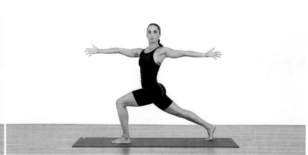

High Lunge: Twist (p. 131)
» 60 seconds per side

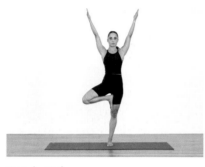

Tree (p. 162)
» 45 seconds per side

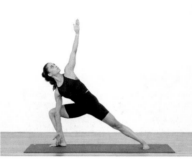

Side Angle (p. 150)
» 30 seconds per side

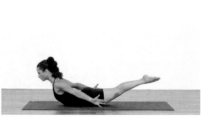

Full Locust (p. 126)
» 30 seconds

RUNNER'S WARM-UP

- Activates key muscles involved in running
- Increases functional mobility to improve performance
- Reduces strain on knees, back, and ankles

Total time: 6 minutes

Hold each posture for the recommended time.
No equipment required
Workout type: Warm-up, standalone

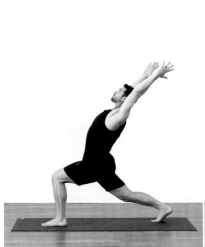

High Lunge: Backbend (p. 131)
» 45 seconds per side

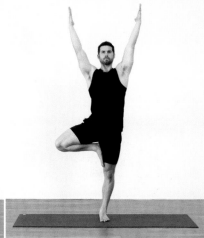

Tree (p. 162)
» 60 seconds per side

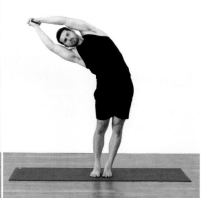

Standing Sidebend (p. 158)
» 30 seconds per side

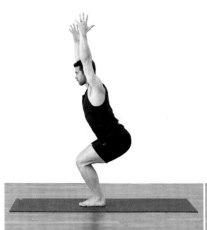

Chair (p. 114)
» 30 seconds

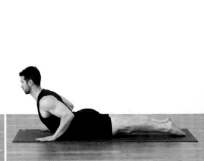

Cobra (p. 118)
» 30 seconds

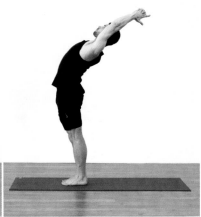

Standing Backbend (p. 154)
» 30 seconds

COMPOUND STRENGTH MOVEMENT WARM-UP

- Full-body routine that prepares body for strong, mobile lifting
- Activates the key muscles in the hips, core, and shoulders involved in compound lifting movements
- Increases functional mobility for the training session
- Improves overall strength potential

Total time: 11 minutes

Hold each posture for the recommended time.

No equipment required

Workout type: Standalone, warm-up

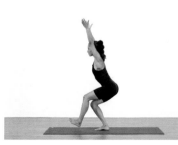

Bridge: Single-Leg (p. 111)
» 30 seconds per side

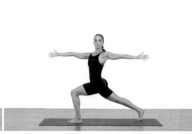

Side Plank (p. 152)
» 45 seconds per side

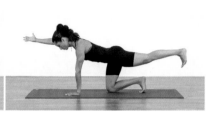

Bird Dog (p. 106)
» 30 seconds per side

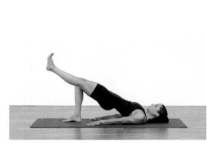

Chair (Single-Leg; optional) (p. 114)
» 60 seconds (or 30 seconds per side)

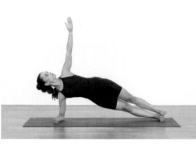

High Lunge: Twist (p. 131)
» 60 seconds per side

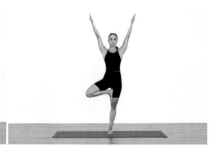

Tree (p. 162)
» 60 seconds per side

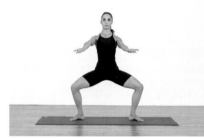

Horse (p. 132)
» 60 seconds

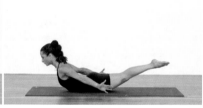

Full Locust or Superman (p. 126)
» 30 seconds

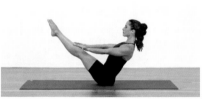

Boat (p. 108)
» 45 seconds

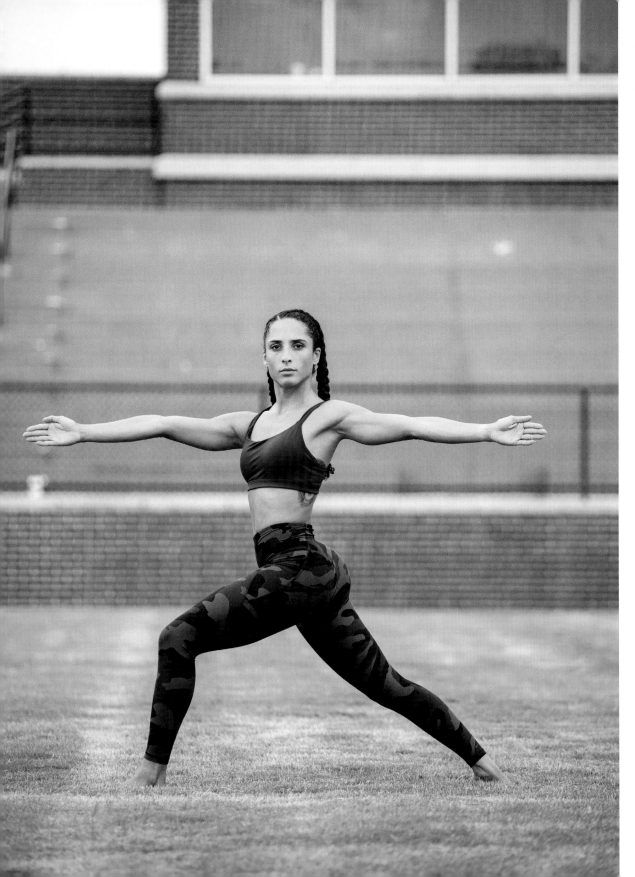

WARM-UP FOR HEALTHY SHOULDERS

- Prepares shoulders for strong, pain-free exercise with a combination of mobility and strength work
- Targets core, hips, and back
- Corrects postural imbalances from inactivity

Total time: 9 minutes
Hold each posture for the recommended time.
Equipment: Strap
Workout type: Warm-up, standalone

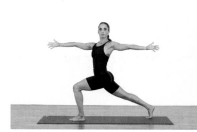

Side Plank (p. 152)
» 45 seconds per side

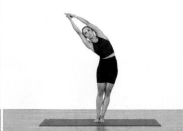

Standing Sidebend (p. 158)
» 30 seconds per side

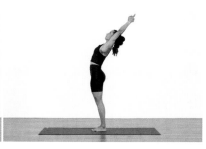

Standing Backbend (p. 154)
» 30 seconds

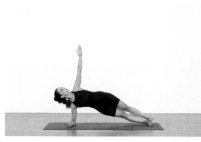

High Lunge: Twist (p. 131)
» 45 seconds per side

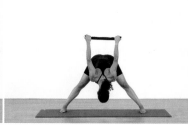

Wide-Legged Forward Fold: With Strap (p. 171)
» 60 seconds

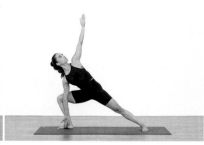

Side Angle (p. 150)
» 30 seconds per side

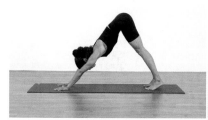

Downdog (p. 122)
» 60 seconds

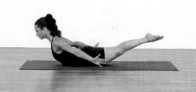

Full Locust (p. 126)
» 30 seconds

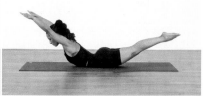

Superman (p. 127)
» 30 seconds

KNEE SORENESS RELIEF

- Stretches muscles in the lower body to relieve tension on the knees
- Targets hips, thighs, and lower legs
- Speeds up recovery and decreases risk of overtraining injuries

Total time: 9 minutes

Hold each posture for the recommended time.

Equipment: Block, strap

Workout type: Standalone, cooldown, restorative

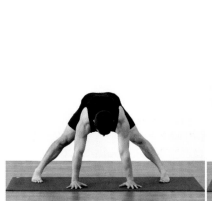

Wide-Legged Forward Fold (p. 170)
» 60 seconds

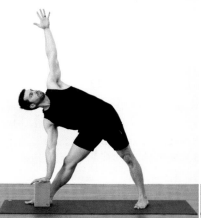

Triangle: Supported on Block (p. 165)
» 45 seconds per side

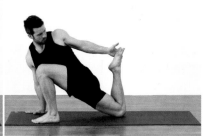

Lizard (Reachback; optional) (p. 134)
» 45 seconds per side

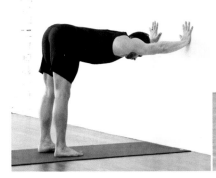

Downdog (On Wall; optional) (p. 122)
» 45 seconds

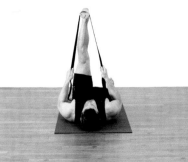

Hamstring Strap Stretch (p. 142)
» 60 seconds per side

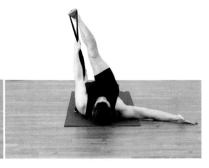

Abductor Strap Stretch (p. 143)
» 60 seconds per side

UPPER-BODY & SHOULDER SORENESS RELIEF

- Relieves muscle tightness in the chest, upper back, arms, and shoulders
- Relieves joint pain in the shoulders, elbows, or wrists
- Helps relieve headaches and neck pain

Total time: 10 minutes

Hold each posture for the recommended time.

Required Equipment: Blocks, strap

Workout type: Standalone, cooldown, restorative

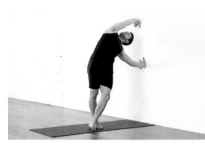

Standing Sidebend: On Wall (p. 159)
» 45 seconds per side

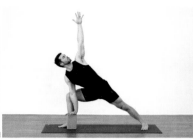

Side Angle: Supported on Block (p. 151)
» 45 seconds per side

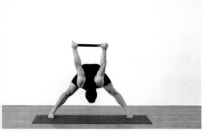

Wide-Legged Forward Fold: With Strap (p. 171)
» 60 seconds

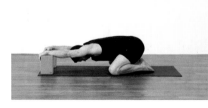

Child's Pose: Supported on Blocks (p. 116)
» 90 seconds

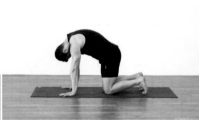

Cat-Cow (p. 112)
» 5–10 reps

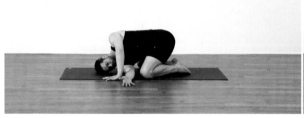

Thread the Needle (p. 160)
» 60 seconds per side

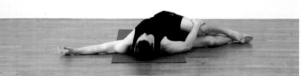

Reclined Twist (p. 144)
» 45 seconds per side

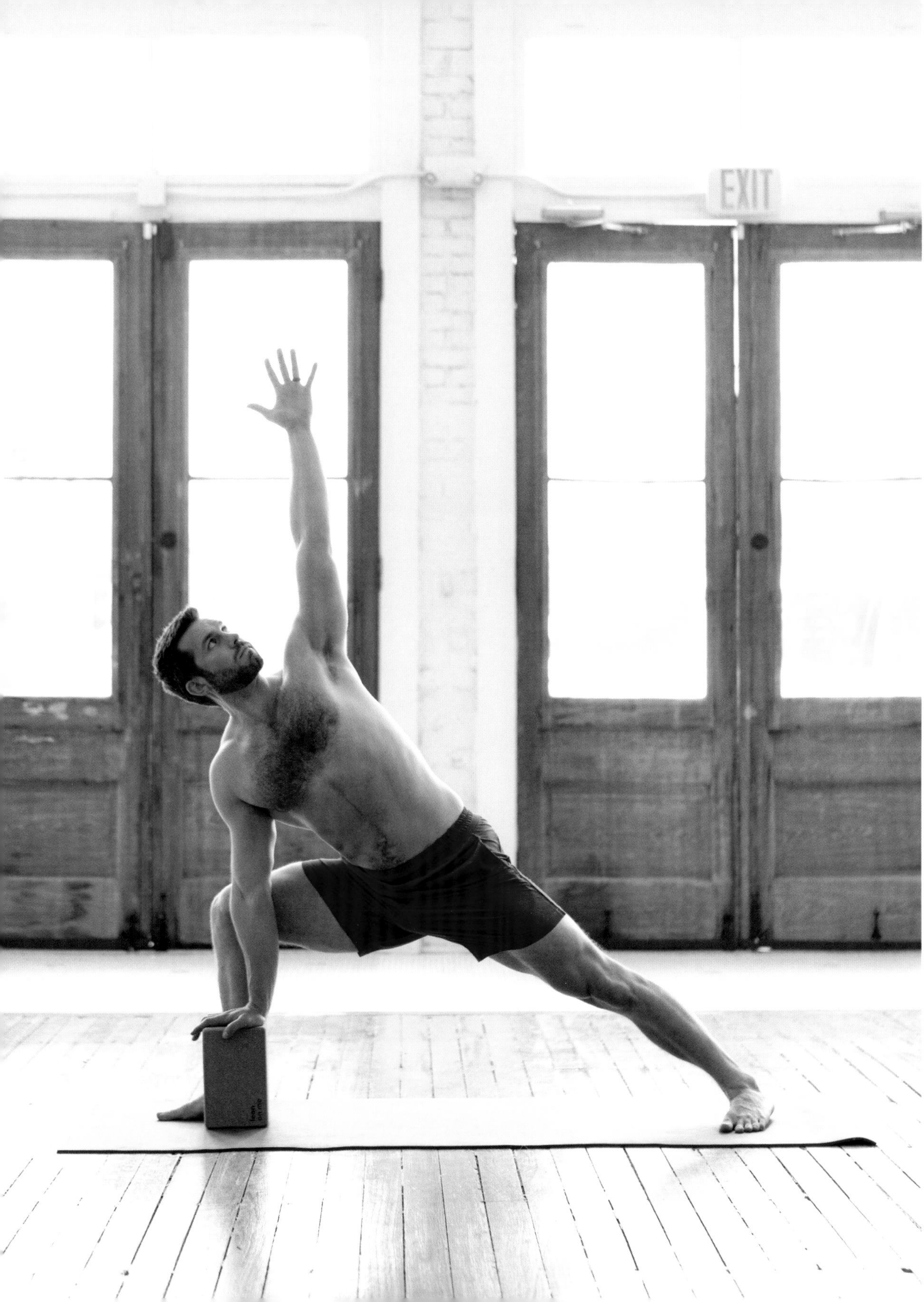
EXIT

BACK PAIN RELIEF

- Relieves back pain with a combination of strengthening and stretching
- Targets root causes of back pain
- Strengthens and stretches hips, core, and back

Total time: 10 minutes

Hold each posture for the recommended time.

No equipment required

Workout type: Restorative, standalone

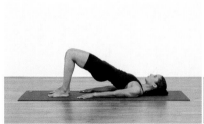

Child's Pose (p. 116)
» 60 seconds

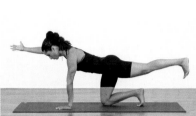

Bird Dog (p. 106)
» 30 seconds per side

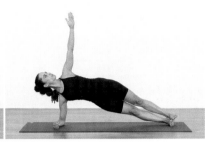

Side Plank (p. 152)
» 30 seconds per side

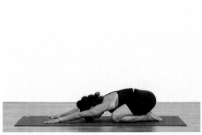

Bridge (p. 110)
» 45 seconds

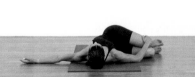

Reclined Twist (p. 144)
» 30 seconds per side

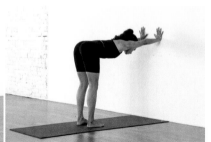

Downdog: On Wall (p. 123)
» 60 seconds

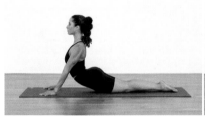

Cobra: Supported (p. 119)
» 30 seconds

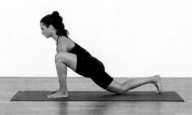

Lizard (p. 134)
» 60 seconds per side

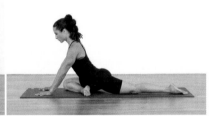

Pigeon (p. 138)
» 60 seconds per side

TOTAL SPINE RELIEF

- Stretches muscles connected to the spine (depending on your back pain, some of these postures may feel better than others, so choose the ones that feel good, and avoid the ones that cause significant discomfort)
- Stretches hips, back, shoulders, and neck
- Increases hip and back flexibility

Total time: 8 minutes

Hold each posture for the recommended time.

No equipment required

Workout type: Standalone, cooldown, restorative

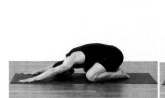

Child's Pose (p. 116)
» 90 seconds

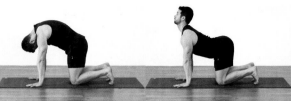

Cat-Cow (p. 112)
» 5–10 reps

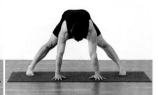

Wide-Legged Forward Fold (p. 170)
» 45 seconds

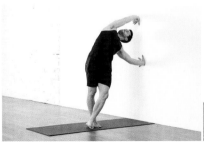

Standing Sidebend: On Wall (p. 159)
» 30 seconds per side

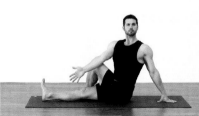

Seated Twist (p. 148)
» 30 seconds per side

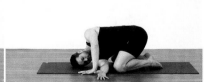

Thread the Needle (p. 160)
» 30 seconds per side

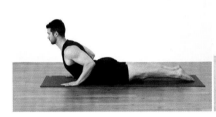

Cobra (p. 118)
» 30 seconds

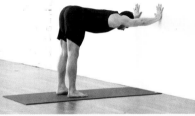

Downdog (On Wall; optional) (p. 122)
» 45 seconds

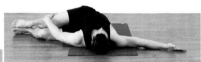

Reclined Twist (p. 144)
» 30 seconds per side

FULL-BODY RESTORATION

- Full-body, full-length workout that releases muscle tightness and joint tension
- Increases flexibility
- Speeds up recovery
- Great for off-days or after a workout

Total time: 18 minutes
Hold each posture for the recommended time.
Equipment: Block, strap
Workout type: Standalone, cooldown, restorative

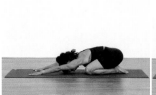

Child's Pose (p. 116)
» 60 seconds

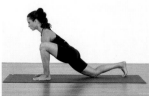

Lizard (p. 134)
» 60 seconds per side

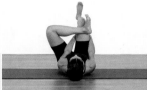

Pigeon or Reclined Figure 4 (p. 138)
» 60 seconds per side

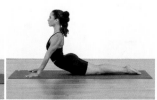

Cobra: Supported (p. 119)
» 30 seconds

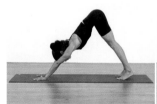

Downdog (On Wall; optional) (p. 122)
» 45 seconds

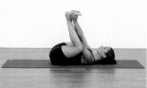

Happy Baby (p. 128)
» 30 seconds

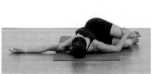

Reclined Twist (p. 144)
» 30 seconds per side

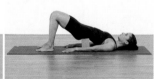

Bridge: Supported on Block (p. 111)
» 60 seconds

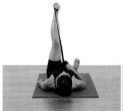

Hamstring Strap Stretch (p. 142)
» 60 seconds per side

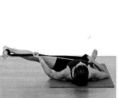

Adductor Strap Stretch (p. 143)
» 60 seconds per side

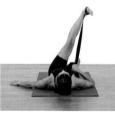

Abductor Strap Stretch (p. 143)
» 60 seconds per side

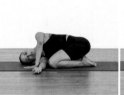

Thread the Needle (p. 160)
» 45 seconds per side

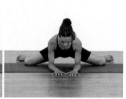

Frog (p. 124)
» 2 minutes

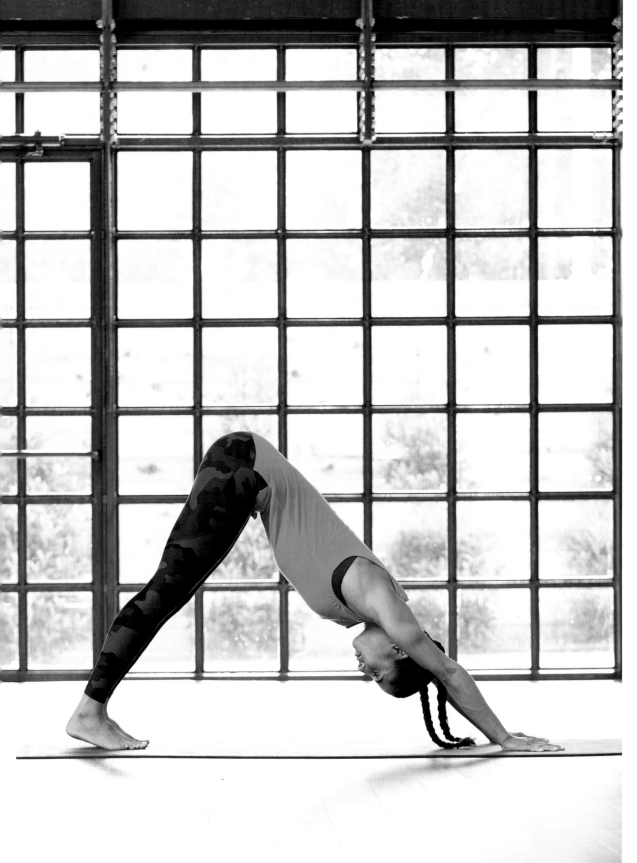

TARGETED WORKOUTS 《《《

101

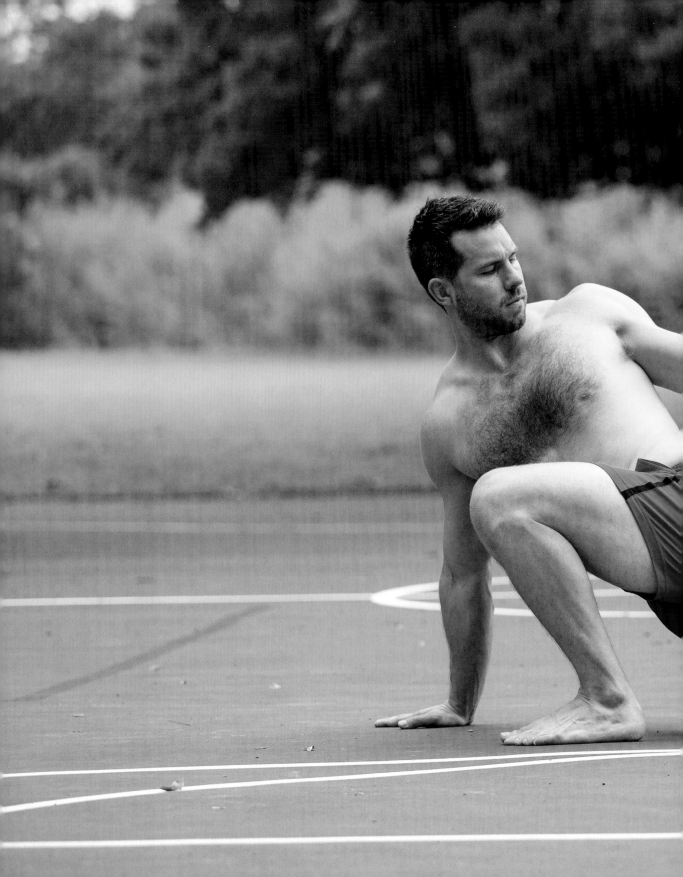

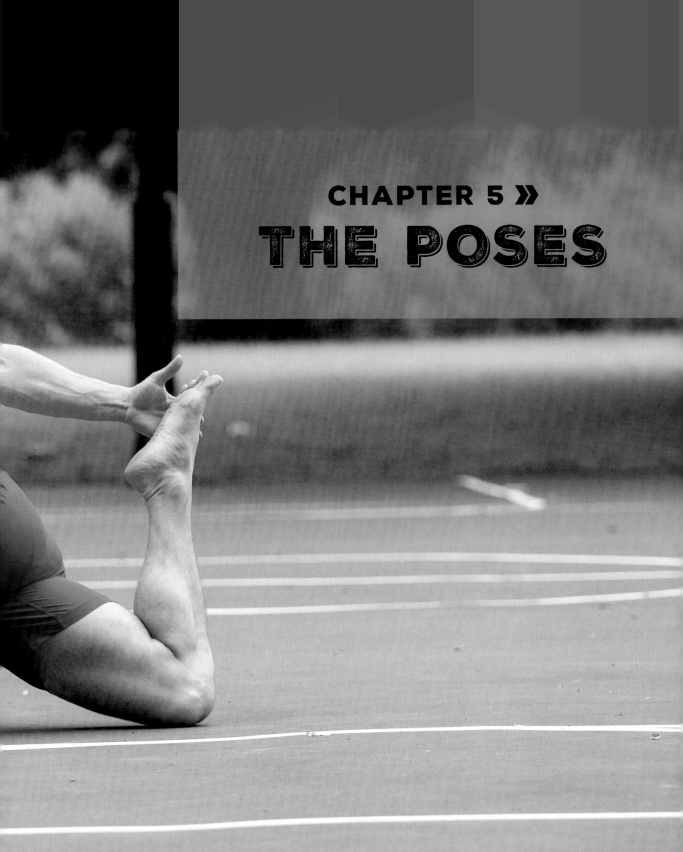

CHAPTER 5 »
THE POSES

AIRPLANE

- Prevents injury in the spine, shoulders, hips, and ankles
- Builds strength and corrects muscular imbalances in the shoulders, upper back, core, hips, and ankles
- Increases flexibility and mobility in the shoulders, hips, hamstrings, and ankles
- Perfect for building core strength and improving balance

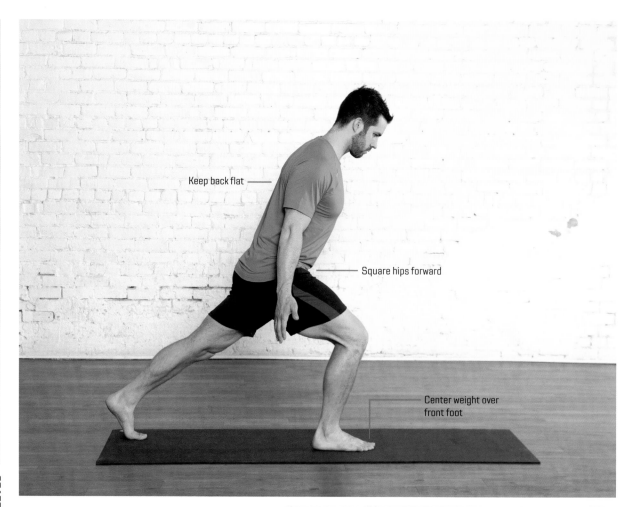

Keep back flat

Square hips forward

Center weight over front foot

1 Stand in a shallow lunge with your hips squared forward and your arms along your sides, palms facing forward.

BUILD STRENGTH IN END RANGE: *To build active mobility in your hips, use only your hips and core (not supporting your hands on the ground or a block) to keep a straight line from your lifted leg through your torso. Point your toes as much as possible to work on foot flexibility and build active ankle mobility.*

2 Maintaining a straight spine with your core engaged, shift your weight into your front foot, and then lift your back leg off the ground, hinging at the hips as you bring your torso forward while extending your back leg. Maintain a straight line from your leg to your head. Keep your arms along your sides. Keep your core actively engaged, and gaze straight down or slightly forward for balance.

Lengthen your body as much as possible, pressing the crown of your head forward, locking out your lifted leg, and pointing your toes. Try to form a T-shape with your body. Work deeper into your hamstrings by straightening your standing leg, but only if your back remains flat. (Most people will have that knee bent.) Inhale to lengthen your spine. Exhale to work deeper into your hip mobility while squeezing your quadriceps.

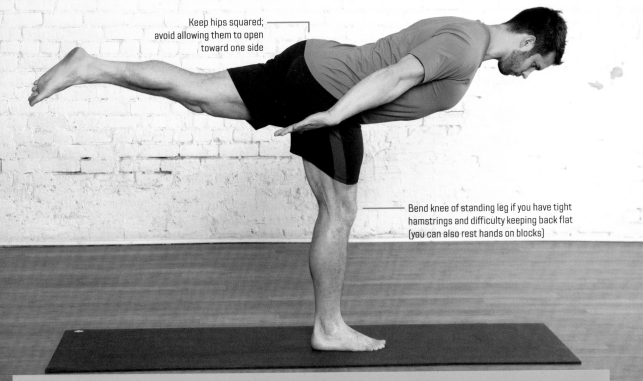

Keep hips squared; avoid allowing them to open toward one side

Bend knee of standing leg if you have tight hamstrings and difficulty keeping back flat (you can also rest hands on blocks)

» VARIATIONS

SUPPORTED ON BLOCKS

For: an emphasis on hamstring mobility or to help develop balance

Place blocks directly under your shoulders and rest hands on them. Bend your knees if necessary, and keep your back flat. Consider stacking blocks on top of one another if hamstrings are extra tight.

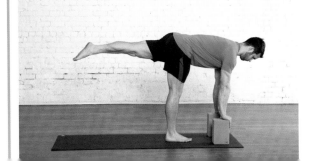

WARRIOR 3

For: a more advanced version

This is a full-body, active mobility–focused version of Airplane. Interlace your fingers and extend your arms overhead, forming a T-shape with your body. If your shoulders are tight, use a strap to hold your hands at shoulder width.

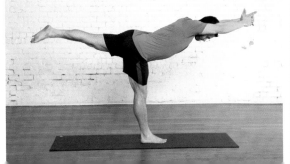

BIRD DOG

- Prevents injury in the spine, shoulders, knees, and hips
- Builds strength and corrects muscular imbalances in the spine, core, hips, and shoulders
- Increases flexibility and mobility in the shoulders, hips, and ankles
- Perfect as a warm-up: targeted core activation, hip strength and awareness, ankle mobility, and shoulder opening

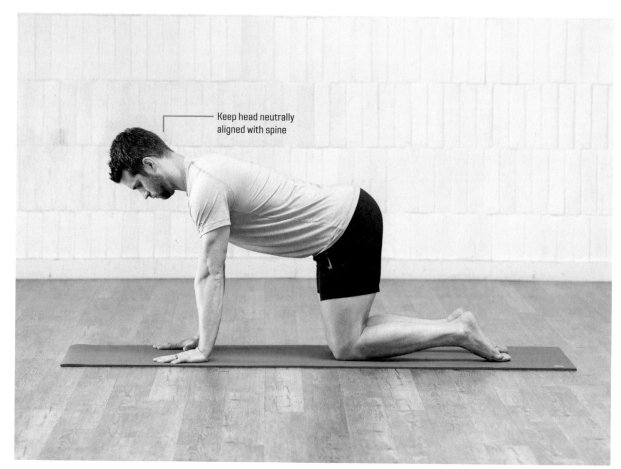

Keep head neutrally aligned with spine

1 Start in a tabletop position with your hips stacked over your knees and your shoulders stacked over your hands. Keep your spine and neck neutral and look straight down. Lightly engage your core. Untuck your toes.

BUILD STRENGTH IN END RANGE: *Actively stretch your heel as far back as possible, and squeeze your raised arm as high as possible (while not arching your back) to build strength in your ankles and shoulders.*

BRIAN'S BREATHING HINT: *Keep your chin neutral; if you notice that your breath is restricted through the neck, then lengthen your neck.*

Press hand forward
and upward
Keep core engaged
(don't let lower back arch)
Keep hip of lifted leg down
(don't let it open up to the side)
Focus gaze straight down
Plant fist instead of palm
if you have pain in wrist
(you can also try holding a
push-up bar or dumbbell)
Keep foot
actively flexed

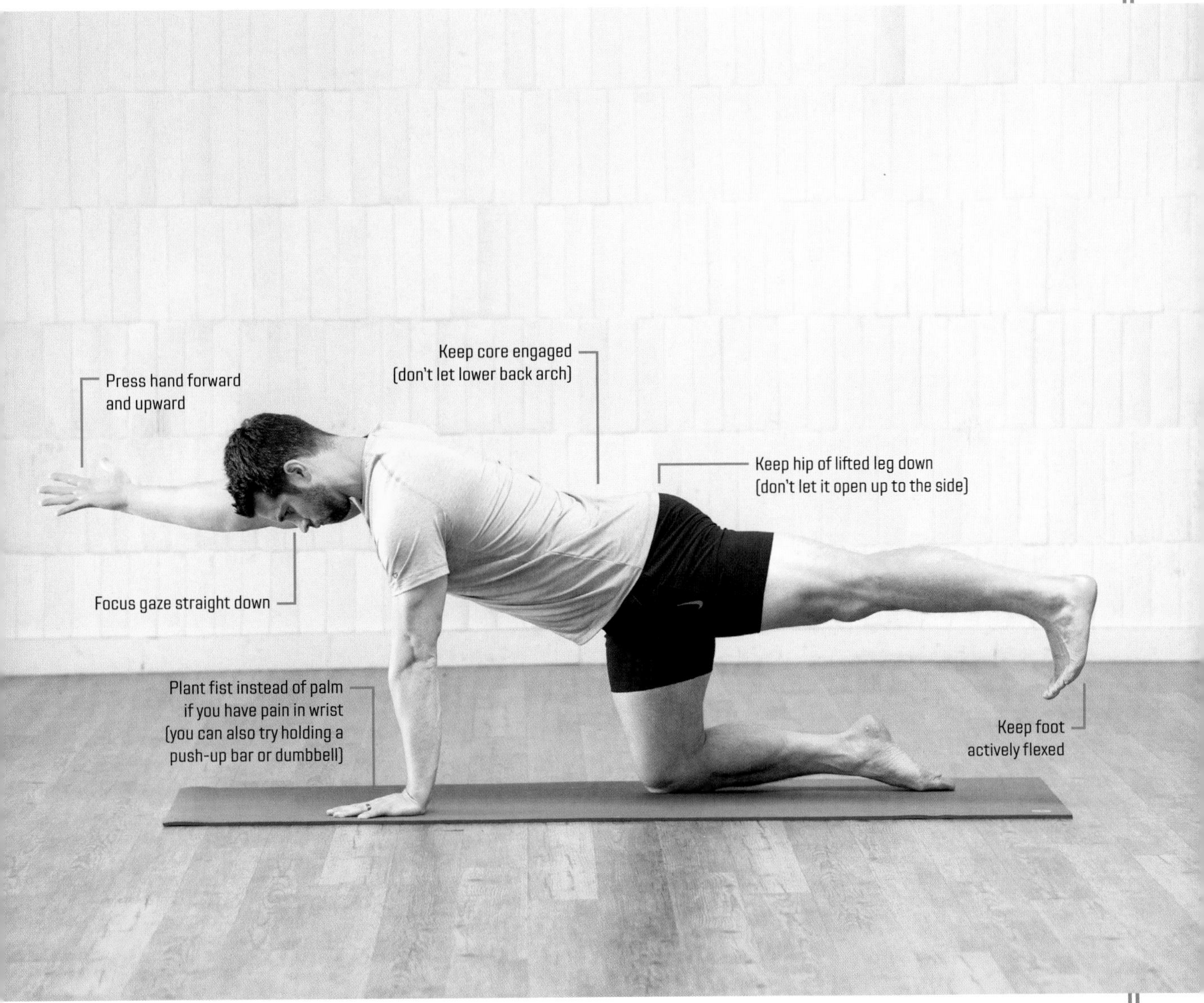

2 Without moving the rest of your body, extend one arm forward to form a straight line from your hips to your extended fingertips, biceps facing your ear. (You should not be able to see your arm.) Then extend your opposite leg straight back, toes flexed toward your shin and heel pressing as far back as possible, forming a straight line from your heel to your extended fingertips. Internally rotate your lifted thigh to keep your hips square to the ground. Inhale to lengthen your neck, and exhale to pull your ribcage toward the top of your abs.

When finished, slowly return your extended arm and leg to the tabletop position. Repeat on the other side.

BOAT

- Prevents injury in the spine, hips, knees, and shoulders
- Builds strength and corrects muscular imbalances in the core and hips
- Increases flexibility and mobility in the hips
- Perfect for building overall core and hip strength

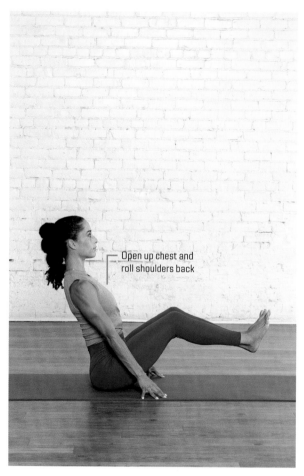

Open up chest and roll shoulders back

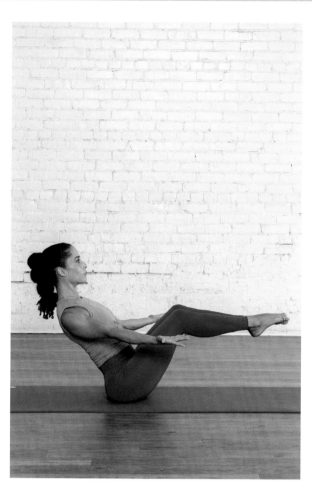

1 Start in a seated position, with your feet planted in front of you and your knees bent. Place your hands on either side of your hips, sit as upright as possible, and lean back slightly to point your chest upward and straighten your spine. Slowly lift your feet off the floor. If your back rounds and your chest caves in, you may grab your knees or keep your hands on the floor to help support yourself in an upright position.

2 Keeping your chest lifted and your back neutral (not rounded), lift your shins parallel to the floor. Engage your hip flexors and quadriceps to hold yourself upright, and extend your arms in front of you, palms facing up. Inhale to lift your chest and maintain upright posture. Exhale to squeeze your core, tighten your quadriceps, and increase overall muscle activation. Stay in this position, or move to step 3 if you're able.

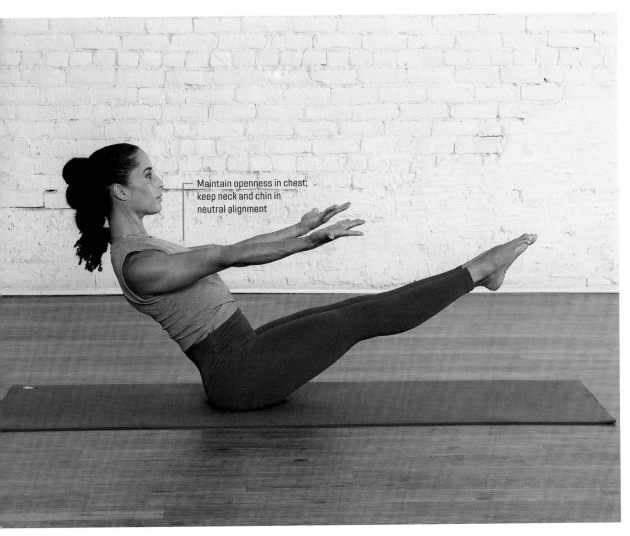

Maintain openness in chest; keep neck and chin in neutral alignment

BUILD STRENGTH IN END RANGE: *Squeeze your quadriceps and hip flexors to further extend your knees and build active mobility in your hamstrings.*

3 To go further, straighten your legs as much as possible while maintaining a straight spine. (If your back starts rounding and your chest caves in, or if your hamstrings are too tight, don't straighten your legs as much, or revert to step 2.) Keep your chest lifting toward the ceiling. Keep your hip flexors, quadriceps, and abs extremely active. Continue to breathe.

BRIDGE

- Prevents injury in the spine, hips, knees, and ankles
- Builds strength and corrects muscular imbalances in the hips, core, and spine
- Increases flexibility and mobility in the hips
- Perfect for developing glute strength and awareness

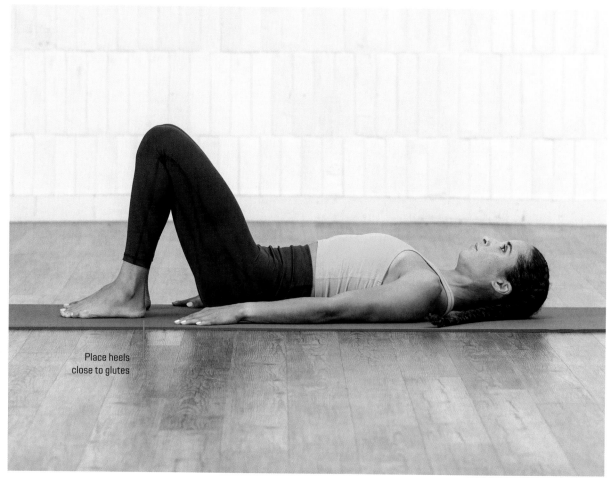

Place heels close to glutes

1 Lie on your back with your arms at your sides. Keep your shoulders, head, and neck relaxed. Plant your feet hip width apart, knees bent, placing your heels just in front of your hips. Point your toes straight forward.

BUILD STRENGTH IN END RANGE: *Strengthen the hamstrings and build active mobility by "pulling" your upper body forward using your feet, and contract your hamstrings as much as you can (while keeping the spine neutral, not arched).*

2 Press your feet into the floor. Engage your core and squeeze your glutes to lift your hips, making sure to keep your spine neutral (not arched). Focus on engaging your glutes and hips. If your back arches, you may be pressing your hips too high. Inhale as you lift your hips higher, and exhale to tighten your core.

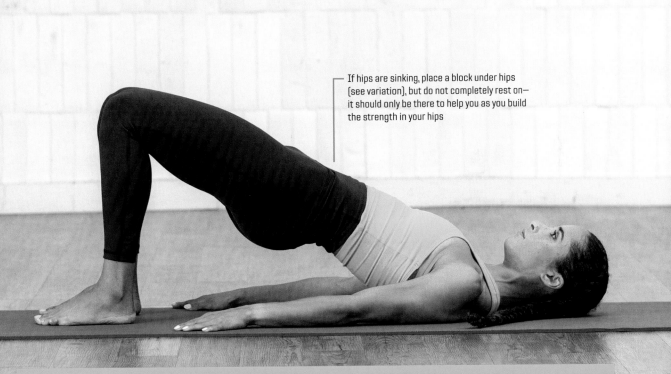

If hips are sinking, place a block under hips (see variation), but do not completely rest on— it should only be there to help you as you build the strength in your hips

» VARIATIONS

SINGLE-LEG

For: building glute strength and hip stability

Starting from the bridge position (step 2) and keeping your hips squared, slowly extend one leg forward to hover off the ground. Keep your hips facing straight up; avoid allowing the hip of your lifted leg to dip. (You may notice cramping here initially—that's normal. As your hips strengthen over time, the cramps will go away.)

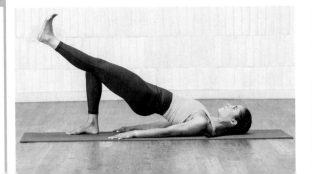

SUPPORTED ON BLOCK

For: a restorative focus/gentle backbend

Place a block just above the sacrum under the lower back, and allow your back to rest there while you breathe. This is great for after any activity when your back may have been in a compromised, flexed position, such as a dead lift or other bent-over exercise, or from activities that involve extended periods of sitting.

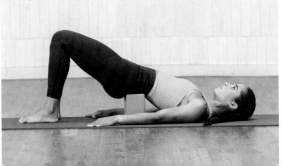

CAT-COW

- Prevents injury in the spine and shoulders
- Builds strength and corrects muscular imbalances in the shoulders, upper back, and spine
- Increases flexibility and mobility in the spine
- Perfect for overall mobility of the spine, as well as for warm-up or recovery

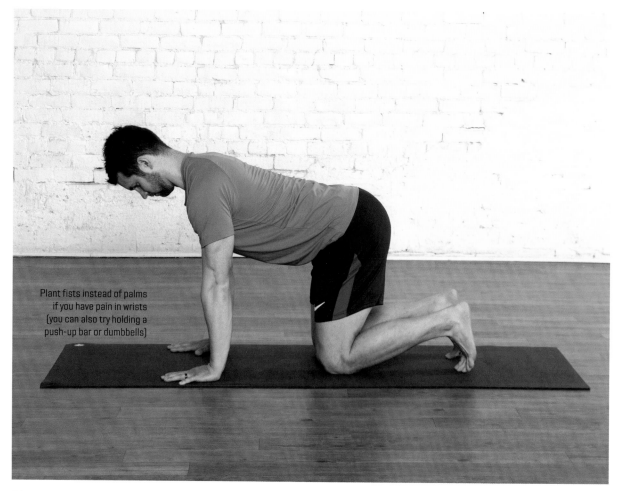

Plant fists instead of palms if you have pain in wrists (you can also try holding a push-up bar or dumbbells)

1 Start in a tabletop position with your hips stacked over your knees and your shoulders stacked over your hands. Keep your spine and neck neutral and look straight down at the floor. Lightly engage your core. Tuck your toes.

BUILD STRENGTH IN END RANGE: For Cat, squeeze the muscles in your core to work deeper into your active spinal flexion. For Cow, squeeze the muscles in your back to work deeper into the active spinal extension.

BRIAN'S BREATHING HINT: *Wait until the very end of the inhale or exhale to fully flex or extend your neck—you shouldn't feel your breath get caught in your throat. You can adjust your breathing on the next inhale/exhale cycle.*

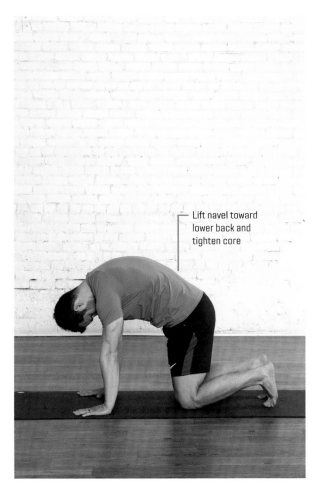

Lift navel toward lower back and tighten core

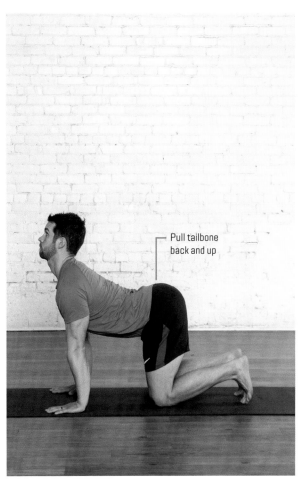

Pull tailbone back and up

2 Cat: Exhale to squeeze your abdominals and transition to a rounded, or flexed, spine. Tuck your chin, separate your shoulder blades, and reach your tailbone down to round your entire spine.

3 Cow: Inhale to arch or extend your entire spine, pulling your chest forward and up, bringing your shoulder blades together, and lifting your tailbone toward the ceiling. Maintain length in your spine as you arch; don't allow your back or your neck to collapse.

Guided by the tempo of your breath, move back and forth from Cat to Cow. You might not be able to keep all technique points in mind the first few times; focus initially on matching Cow to your inhale and Cat to your exhale.

CHAIR

- Prevents injury in the back, hips, knees, ankles, and shoulders
- Builds strength and corrects muscular imbalances in the hips, core, ankles, shoulders, and upper back
- Increases flexibility and mobility in the hips, shoulders, and ankles
- Perfect for building hip and core strength, increasing mobility for shoulder flexion, and strengthening the knees and ankles

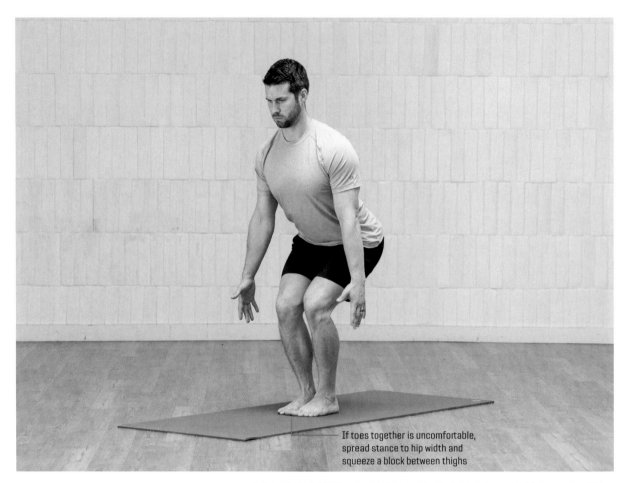

If toes together is uncomfortable, spread stance to hip width and squeeze a block between thighs

1 Stand in Mountain (p. 136) with your big toes nearly touching and your heels about 1 inch (2.5cm) apart. Hinge at your hips and bend your knees to lower your hips, as if you were sitting into a chair, while maintaining a straight spine.

BUILD STRENGTH IN END RANGE: *Without arching your back, squeeze your arms as far back as possible to build more active mobility in your upper back and shoulders. When you maintain proper alignment in your spine, your weight in your hips, and your heels down, you can bend deeper into your knees to increase active mobility in your ankles.*

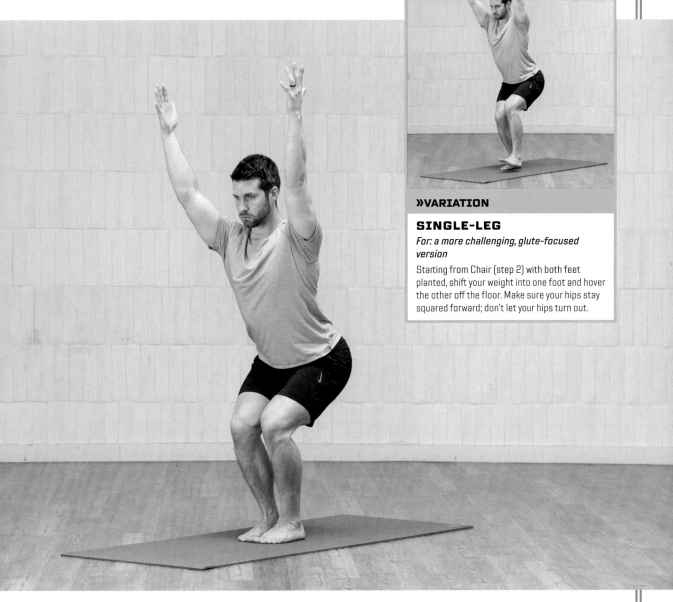

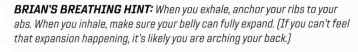

»VARIATION

SINGLE-LEG

For: a more challenging, glute-focused version

Starting from Chair (step 2) with both feet planted, shift your weight into one foot and hover the other off the floor. Make sure your hips stay squared forward; don't let your hips turn out.

2 Maintaining the squat, reach your arms overhead, palms facing each other or turning backward. Continue to hinge at your hips and bend your knees to lower your hips as low as you can while keeping your heels down and your spine neutral. Keep the majority of the weight in your hips (not in your knees). Inhale to maintain length in your spine and hold an upright posture. Exhale to lower yourself deeper into the chair position.

CHILD'S POSE

- Prevents injury in the spine and shoulders
- Corrects muscular imbalances in the upper back and core
- Increases flexibility in the hips, shoulders, and ankles
- Improves focus, realigns the spine, and helps you wind down

NICK'S TIP: *Child's pose is one exercise I really enjoy doing in the morning about 30 minutes or so before a run. The flexibility Child's Pose brings to my shoulders, chest, and upper back is critical to ensuring I have proper breathing mechanics during my tougher, longer runs.*

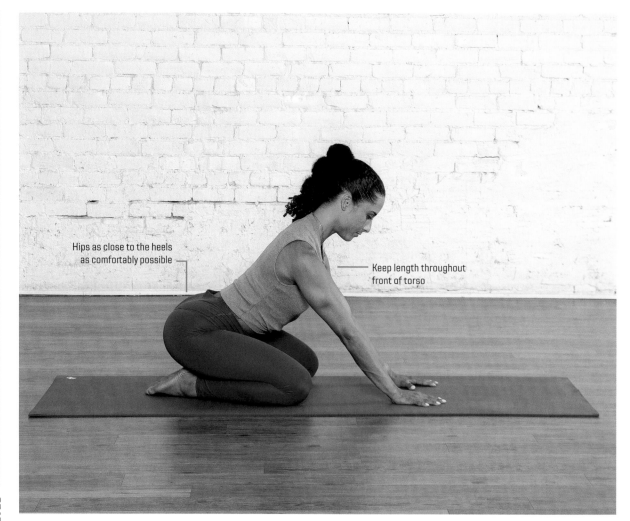

Hips as close to the heels as comfortably possible

Keep length throughout front of torso

1 Start in a kneeling position with your knees spread slightly wider than shoulder-width apart and your big toes touching, feet untucked. Sit your hips back toward your heels. Rest your hands in front of you on the mat.

BUILD STRENGTH IN END RANGE: *Squeeze your arms upward as if you are lifting your hands off the ground, and squeeze your arms toward one another. This engages the scapular stabilizers of your upper back and increases active shoulder mobility.*

BRIAN'S BREATHING HINT: *As you inhale, feel your ribs expand against your chest and the stretch in your chest intensify, breathe into your thoracic spine while maintaining the slight contraction of your transverse abdominals, and lengthen your neck and arms. As you exhale, squeeze your core to exhale completely. You should notice the changing stretch in the upper body surrounding your armpits as you breathe.*

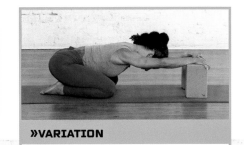

»VARIATION

SUPPORTED ON BLOCKS

For: a deeper shoulder stretch or if you have rounded posture or tight shoulders

Elevate your hands on blocks to further open your shoulders. This helps prevent rounding of the back and increases upper-back engagement. Note that your head may come off the ground—this is fine.

Keep back as flat as possible

Relax head (or rest forehead on a block)

If feet start to cramp, you can tuck toes (but work toward keeping toes untucked)

If you experience knee pain from the fully flexed position, lift hips some to bend knees less

2 Keeping your spine straight and your hips pushed back, fold forward and walk your hands forward at shoulder width to bring your chest and head toward the ground and create a stretch in your shoulders and upper back. Lock out your arms and press your chest toward the floor, keeping your spine neutral (not arched or rounded). Inhale to expand your chest, and exhale to tighten your abs and draw your ribs in.

COBRA

- Prevents injury in the spine, hips, and shoulders
- Builds strength and corrects muscular imbalances in the core, hips, and spine
- Increases flexibility and mobility in the spine and ankles
- Perfect for strengthening the spine and addressing the root causes of back pain

FRANCHESKA'S TIP: *Instead of focusing on how deep you can go in this backbend, prioritize lengthening through your spine and keeping your abdomen and pelvic floor engaged. If you feel limited here, try looking up toward your brow for more range of motion.*

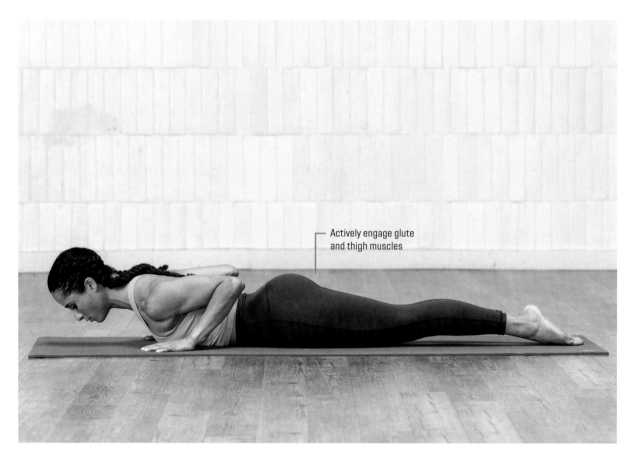

Actively engage glute and thigh muscles

1 Lie on your stomach, and place your hands under your chest with your elbows pointing straight back, upper arms hugged in tight to your sides. Untuck your toes. Internally rotate your thighs so your kneecaps point straight down and the tops of your feet and all toes are touching the floor. Tighten your quadriceps to lift your knees, and squeeze your big toes, ankles, knees, and inner thighs toward each other. Firmly engage your core by squeezing your abdominal wall.

BUILD STRENGTH IN END RANGE: *Continue to press your feet into the ground and squeeze your big toes together. Use only your core strength to maintain height off the ground.*

BRIAN'S BREATHING HINT: *If you notice your inhale is restricted in your throat, then make sure you have proper neck positioning. You should still be feeling your ribs expand in the front, and the focus should be on opening your chest, not your neck. Lastly, acknowledge that this is not a position where you'll be able to breathe normally—and that's okay.*

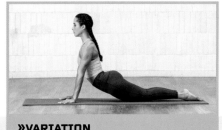

》VARIATION

SUPPORTED

For: a more relaxed flexibility focus

Use your hands to gently assist and press up into a higher Cobra. This opens the chest and strengthens your spine. Avoid overarching and feeling a pinching sensation in your lower back.

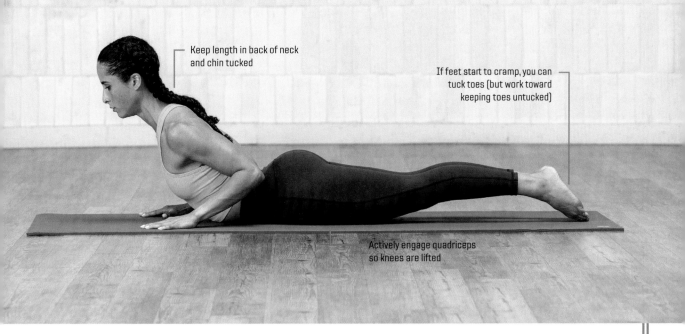

Keep length in back of neck and chin tucked

If feet start to cramp, you can tuck toes (but work toward keeping toes untucked)

Actively engage quadriceps so knees are lifted

2 Inhale to lengthen your spine forward, and then use your core and hip strength to arch your chest away from the floor; don't use your hands to press up. Press the crown of your head away from your shoulders and look slightly forward (and up, if possible). Keep your neck long; avoid collapsing through the back of your neck. Actively retract your shoulder blades by pulling them down and toward one other. Squeeze your elbows tight to your sides, and when you've reached your maximum height, use your hands to pull (not push) your body forward and up. Exhale to maintain the position.

DOLPHIN

- Prevents injury in the shoulders, hips, ankles, and spine
- Builds strength and corrects muscular imbalances in the shoulders, upper back, core, hips, and ankles
- Increases flexibility and mobility in the shoulders, hips, and ankles
- Perfect full-body posture for building upper-back and shoulder strength and mobility

NICK'S TIP: *My shoulders are incredibly tight, so Dolphin is a pose I rely on regularly for my shoulders. Rather than holding it passively, I like to rock back and forth to help mobilize my shoulders and work deeper into the stretch. This is a pose I'll use prerun that, in addition to my shoulders, helps with warming up my hamstrings and calves.*

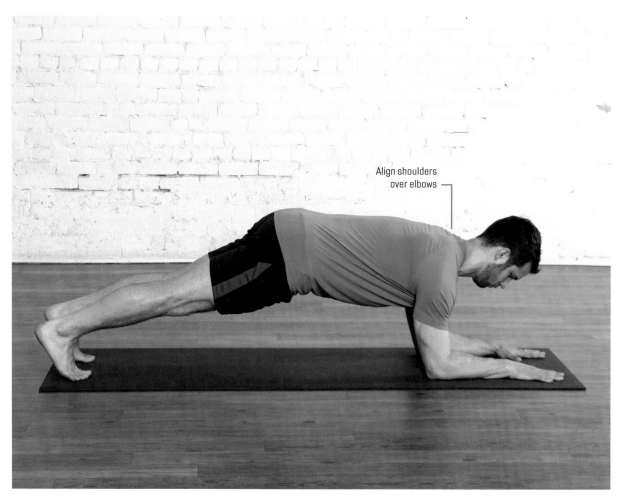

Align shoulders over elbows

1 Start in a forearm plank with your forearms parallel to one another at shoulder width, toes tucked, and knees lifted.

BUILD STRENGTH IN END RANGE: *To build active mobility in your upper body, hug your forearms toward one another to keep arms parallel. Press your chest back to open your shoulders and further engage the muscles in the upper back. To build active mobility in your hips, squeeze your quadriceps and hip flexors. To build active mobility in your ankles, press the tops of your feet and your shins toward one another.*

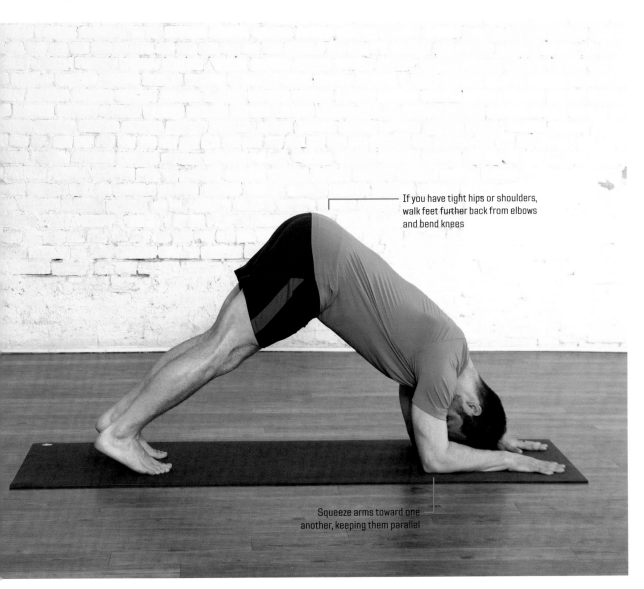

If you have tight hips or shoulders, walk feet further back from elbows and bend knees

Squeeze arms toward one another, keeping them parallel

2 Hike up your hips as you walk your feet in toward your elbows to form a pyramid shape, keeping your back flat. (Bend your knees if your back starts to round.) Reach your tailbone toward the ceiling, engage your quadriceps, and press your hips up and away from your shoulders to lengthen the spine. Press your chest back toward your feet to further open your shoulders. Keep your shoulders above your elbows and your neck relaxed. Squeeze your elbows toward each other. Flex your shins to bring the tops of your feet and shins closer. Inhale to lengthen your spine. Exhale to deepen the stretch in your hamstrings and lats and increase upper-back engagement.

DOWNDOG

- Prevents injury in the spine, shoulders, hips, and ankles
- Builds strength and corrects muscular imbalances in the shoulders, upper back, core, hips, and ankles
- Increases flexibility and mobility in the shoulders, hips, and ankles
- Perfect full-body inversion for practicing proper breathing technique while working on full-body mobility

NICK'S TIP: *I find Downdog mandatory for my entire upper torso—shoulders, midback, upper back, and traps. Doing Downdog before a run prepares me for proper breathing technique, and it also ensures my shoulders stay in a nice, upright position during the run, which in turn supports my neck.*

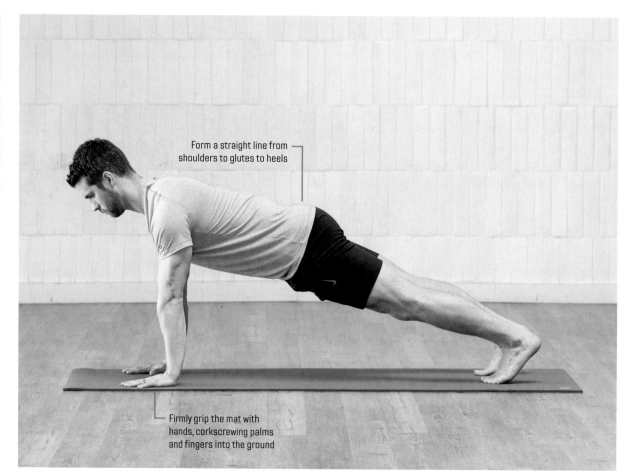

Form a straight line from shoulders to glutes to heels

Firmly grip the mat with hands, corkscrewing palms and fingers into the ground

1 Start in a high plank with your arms extended under your shoulders, toes tucked, and knees lifted.

BUILD STRENGTH IN END RANGE: *For active mobility in your lower body, squeeze your quadriceps, hip flexors, and abs. For active mobility in your upper body, engage the muscles between your shoulder blades to further open your chest.*

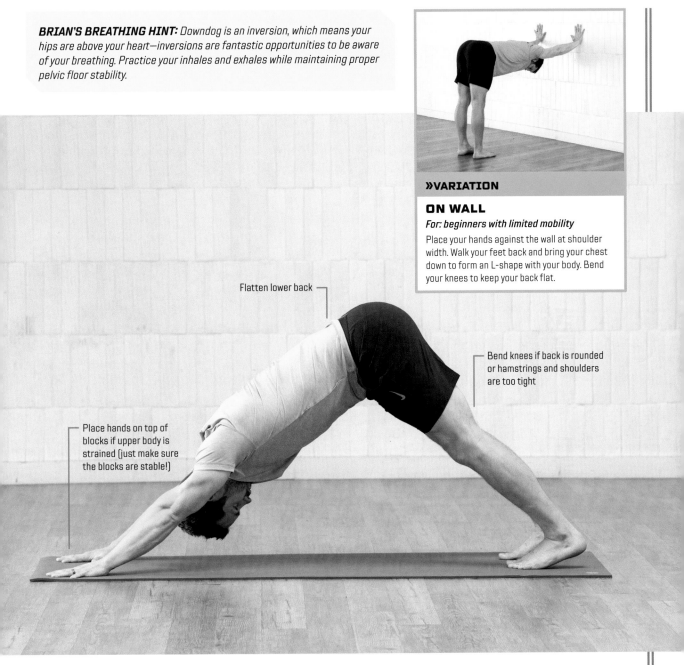

BRIAN'S BREATHING HINT: *Downdog is an inversion, which means your hips are above your heart—inversions are fantastic opportunities to be aware of your breathing. Practice your inhales and exhales while maintaining proper pelvic floor stability.*

»VARIATION

ON WALL
For: beginners with limited mobility
Place your hands against the wall at shoulder width. Walk your feet back and bring your chest down to form an L-shape with your body. Bend your knees to keep your back flat.

Flatten lower back

Bend knees if back is rounded or hamstrings and shoulders are too tight

Place hands on top of blocks if upper body is strained (just make sure the blocks are stable!)

2 Lift your hips up and back to bring your body into a pyramid shape, keeping a straight line from your hips through shoulders and extended arms. Make sure your lower back is neutral, not rounded. Press down firmly through all parts of your hands. Wrap your biceps to face slightly forward. Keep your shoulders down and away from your ears.

Tuck your chin to look back at your feet. Lightly squeeze your quadriceps and core to intensify the hamstring stretch. Flex the tops of your feet toward your shins. Relax your heels to stretch your calves, or actively press your heels toward the floor. Inhale to lengthen and lift. Exhale to stretch deeper into your hamstrings, calves, and shoulders.

FROG

- Prevents injury in the spine, hips, and knees
- Builds strength and corrects muscular imbalances in the hips and spine
- Increases flexibility and mobility in the hips
- Perfect for stretching and increasing overall mobility of the inner thighs (adductors) and excellent for reducing soreness in the hips and knees the day after exercise

FRANCHESKA'S TIP: *If you're looking for more of a challenge and your hips are pretty mobile, turn up the intensity! Rather than going into a passive range of motion, keep your glutes engaged, and gently rock backward and forward.*

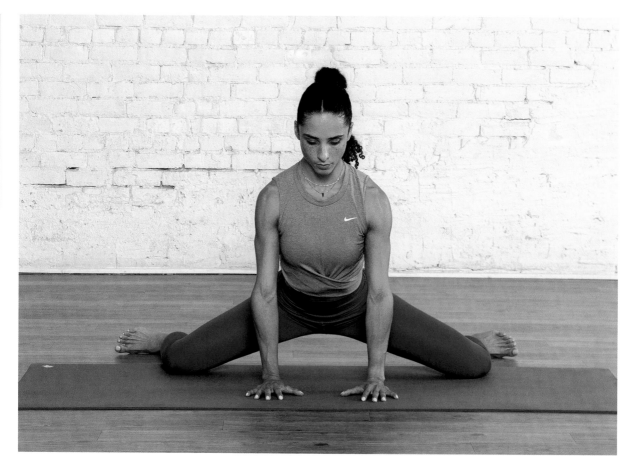

1 Facing the long edge of the mat, get onto all fours and edge your knees outward as far as you comfortably can, noticing the stretch in your inner thighs. (Make sure your knees are comfortable. For added cushion, roll up the narrow edges of the mat and place the folded mat under your knees.) Slide your ankles out to line them up directly under your knees, forming parallel lines with your shins.

BUILD STRENGTH IN END RANGE:
For active mobility in the hips, squeeze your outer glutes to create a deeper stretch. (This pose is already very intense for most people, so you might not need this.)

BRIAN'S BREATHING HINT: *In Frog, the breathing is reverse of what we'd typically do. Spend the first 3 to 5 breaths in this posture using the inhale to relax and the exhale to engage the pelvic floor and adductors. After those initial breaths, focus on completely relaxing the adductors during both the inhale and exhale.*

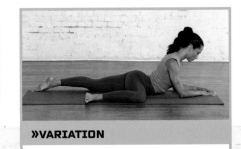

»VARIATION

SINGLE-LEG

For: less intensity

The technique is the same as step 2, but one leg stays bent while the other straightens.

If this stretch is too intense on your hips, try resting your arms on an elevated surface such as a bench or coffee table

2 Form a neutral spine, lightly engage your core (just as you would in Child's Pose or plank), and slowly shift your hips back until you feel a sufficient stretch in the groin. Lower your forearms to the floor. For more intensity, shift your body weight toward your hips. For less intensity, put more of your body weight on your forearms. For many people, this is a very intense hip opener—use your breathing to counter your fight-or-flight response and maintain your composure. Inhale to hold your form. Exhale to relax deeper into the pose and shift hips further back.

FULL LOCUST

- Prevents injury in the spine, shoulders, hips, and ankles
- Builds strength and corrects muscular imbalances in the shoulders, upper back, core, hips, and ankles
- Increases flexibility and mobility in the shoulders, hips, and ankles
- Perfect intense, full-body posture for building strength in the entire posterior chair and core while focusing on active mobility for spinal extension

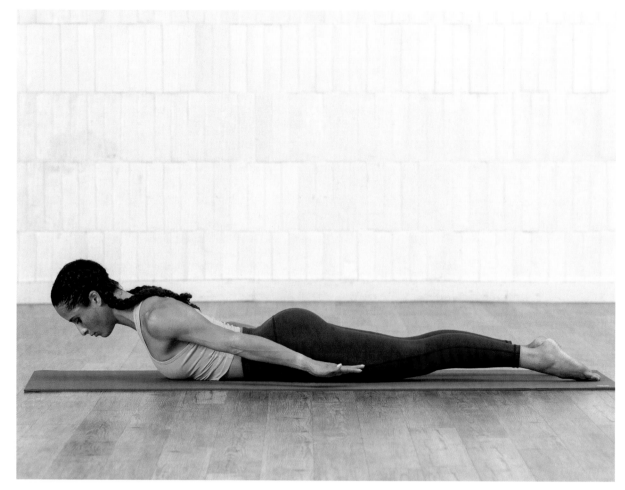

1 Lie on your stomach with your arms flat along your sides, legs extended straight out and toes untucked. Brace your core as you extend your feet as far back as possible, squeezing your quadriceps to lock out your knees. Lift your arms off the floor, keeping your shoulders in an open position.

BUILD STRENGTH IN END RANGE: *When using proper technique, active mobility is already applied in all areas of the body.*

BRIAN'S BREATHING HINT: *The goal here isn't to get as high as possible—it's to get as high as possible* while *maintaining controlled breathing in and out of your nose. Push yourself to go further, but make sure you can maintain a full breath cycle.*

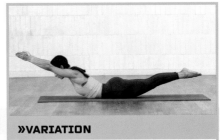

»VARIATION

SUPERMAN

For: a challenging shoulder and upper-back component to an already-intense pose

Extend your arms forward and squeeze them as high as you can. Maintain length from tailbone to crown of head, and avoid craning your neck upward.

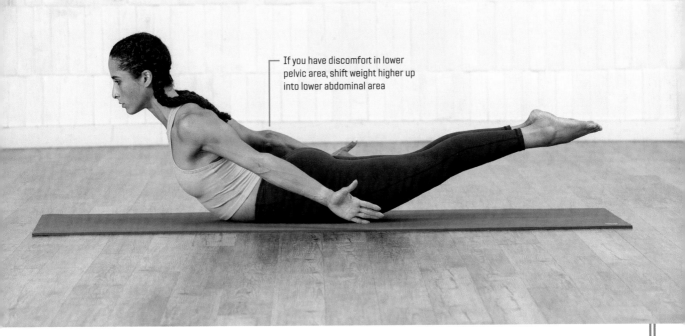

If you have discomfort in lower pelvic area, shift weight higher up into lower abdominal area

2 Once you have fully lengthened your body, lift your legs and your torso to actively arch your back. Squeeze your arms upward to activate the upper-back and rotator-cuff muscles. Maintain intense core and hip engagement for the duration of the pose, taking special care to maintain a strong backbend and keeping length in the lower back and neck. Inhale to lengthen and lift your body. Exhale to extend your toes further back and press the crown of your head forward.

HAPPY BABY

- Prevents injury in the spine, hips, and knees
- Builds strength and corrects muscular imbalances in the hips
- Increases flexibility and mobility in the hips
- Perfect as a non-weight-bearing posture for increasing groin mobility and relieving lower-back stiffness

FRANCHESKA'S TIP: *If you're more flexible, work on getting deeper into this with strength. Inhale to push your feet into your hands. Exhale to pull your knees closer to your chest.*

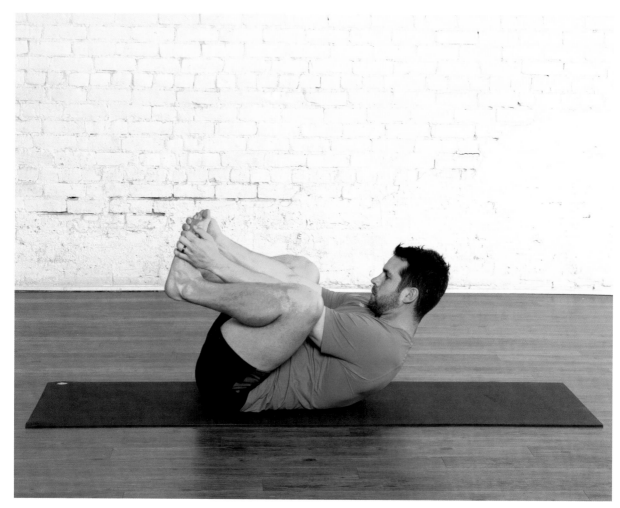

1 Lying on your back, bend your knees in toward your shoulders and grab the outsides of your feet with your hands so your palms are facing one another. Keep your elbows inside your knees, and make sure most of your lower back remains relaxed on the ground.

BUILD STRENGTH IN END RANGE: *Squeeze your hamstrings, inner thighs, and outer thighs. Press your feet up into your hands, and use your hands to pull your feet toward the floor to increase active range of motion in your hips.*

BRIAN'S BREATHING HINT: Use your breathing to ensure your depth is appropriate for your flexibility level. As you inhale, fill your pelvic floor as much as possible—you should be able to feel your pelvic floor expand as you inhale. If you feel restricted, bend your knees more. You can also use a strap around the soles of your feet so your lower spine can fully relax on the ground.

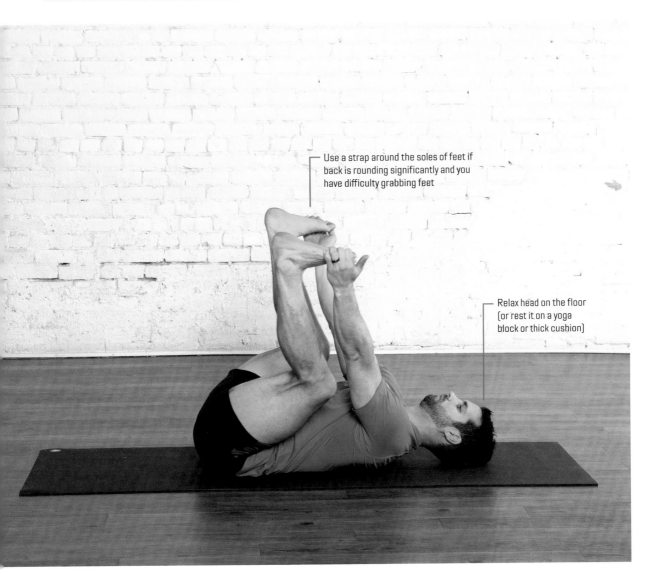

Use a strap around the soles of feet if back is rounding significantly and you have difficulty grabbing feet

Relax head on the floor (or rest it on a yoga block or thick cushion)

2 Relax your shoulders and head on the floor. Flex your toes toward your shins and aim the soles of your feet upward. Drive your knees out and extend your legs until you feel an adequate stretch in your inner thighs, keeping your lower back on the ground as much as possible. Inhale to maintain the position, and exhale to deepen the stretch.

HIGH LUNGE

- Prevents injury in the spine, hips, ankles, and shoulders
- Builds strength and corrects muscle imbalances in the hips, core, ankles, and shoulders
- Increases flexibility and mobility in the hips and shoulders
- Perfect lower-body balance posture to actively open hips and prepare your body for exercise

NICK'S TIP: *High Lunge is a pose that really helps with my hip flexor tightness, which has always been a big pain point for me. I'll use this 30 minutes or so before a run to make sure my hips stay loose.*

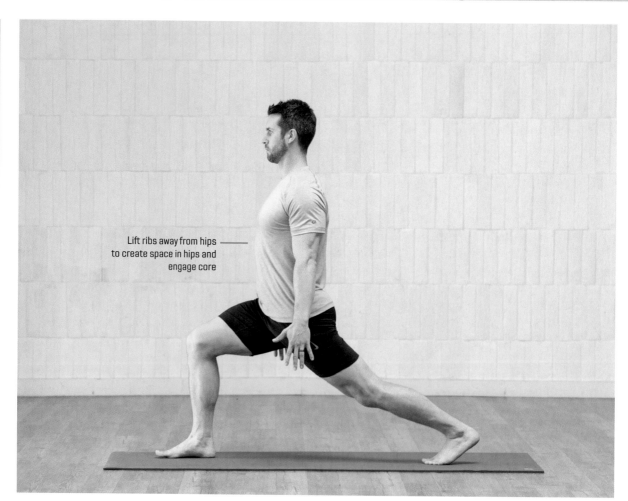

Lift ribs away from hips to create space in hips and engage core

1 Standing at the top of your mat, take a big step back with one foot, and plant the ball of your foot on the ground, heel lifted. Bend your front knee until the shin is perpendicular to the floor. Actively press the entire front foot and toes into the floor, keeping the arch engaged and lifted, as if you are grabbing the ground with your foot.

BUILD STRENGTH IN END RANGE: *To build active mobility in your adductors and hip flexors, squeeze your legs toward one another. To build active mobility in your upper back, squeeze your arms as far back as possible without arching your back.*

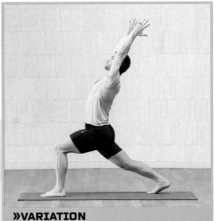

»VARIATION

BACKBEND

For: a deeper hip flexor stretch and spinal extension focus

Keeping hips squared forward and lower back neutral, reach your arms up and back, and lean back into a strong, controlled backbend. Keep neck elongated and maintain proper High Lunge technique with the lower body. Avoid pinching in your lower back.

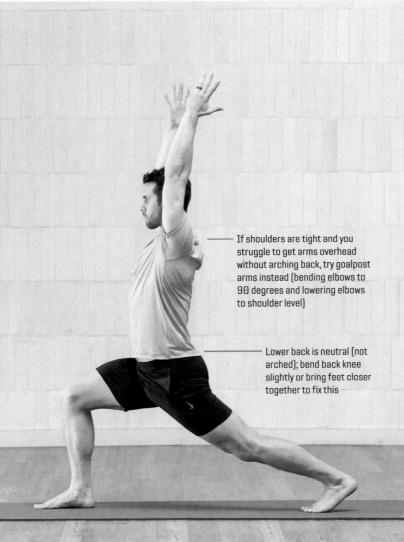

If shoulders are tight and you struggle to get arms overhead without arching back, try goalpost arms instead (bending elbows to 90 degrees and lowering elbows to shoulder level)

Lower back is neutral (not arched); bend back knee slightly or bring feet closer together to fix this

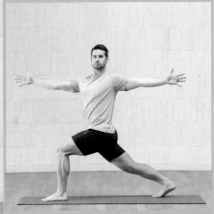

»VARIATION

TWIST

For: a thoracic mobility component

Keeping hips squared forward, rotate from your middle back (thoracic spine) to face sideways, twisting in the direction of the forward leg. Extend your arms to the sides, reaching in opposite directions at shoulder level. You'll feel the muscles in your upper back engage as you hold this. To further isolate thoracic mobility, interlace your fingers behind your neck to focus on the twist in your spine.

2 Reach your arms straight overhead, but avoid puffing out your chest and arching your back. You should feel a stretch in your hip flexors; if you don't, widen your stance or sink deeper into your lunge. Inhale to lengthen the spine and maintain the stance. Exhale to sink deeper into the lunge.

HORSE

- Prevents injury in the knees, hips, and spine
- Builds strength and corrects muscular imbalances in the hips
- Increases flexibility and mobility in the hips
- Perfect for building active mobility in the groin and very effective for reducing exercise strain in the knees and lower back

FRANCHESKA'S TIP: Don't go for depth here. Focus on proper form! Spending time in this pose is great for strengthening the deep muscles of the hips and feet, too.

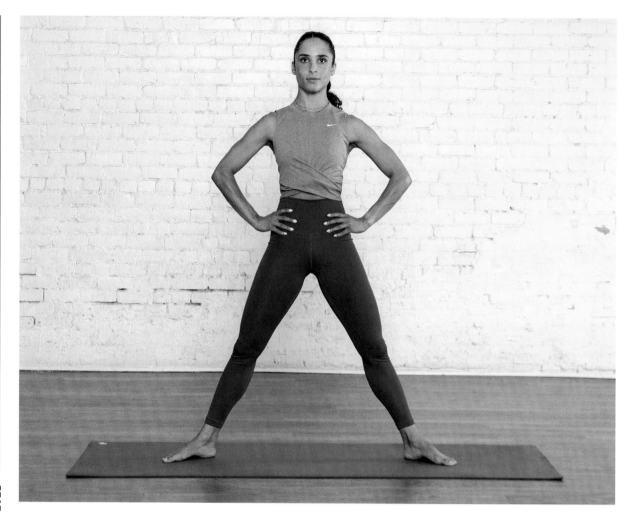

1 Stand with your feet 4 to 5 feet (1.25–1.5m) apart (wider if you are taller) and toes turned out to about 45 degrees. (If your hips are more flexible, you can turn your toes all the way out.)

BUILD STRENGTH IN END RANGE: To build active hip mobility, maintain glute engagement and squeeze your heels toward one another. Use your body weight to sink deeper into the posture and further challenge your mobility.

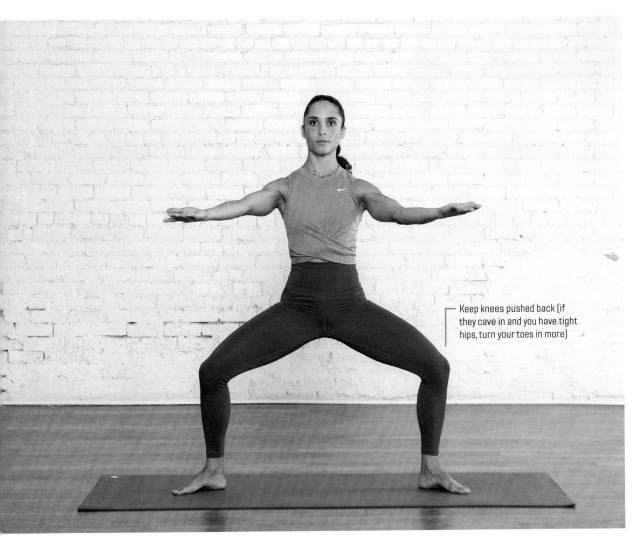

Keep knees pushed back (if they cave in and you have tight hips, turn your toes in more)

2 Sink into a wide-legged squat with your toes pointed out, spine neutral, and knees tracking over your middle toes. (Do not allow your knees or the arches of your feet to cave in.) Firmly engage your glutes, and squeeze your core to keep your hips under your torso, avoiding excessive arching in your lower back. Extend your arms out in front of you to help counterbalance, and go as deep into the squat as you can with neutral spinal alignment. Inhale to check in with your technique and maintain length through the spine. Exhale to sink deeper.

LIZARD

- Prevents injury in the spine, hips, and knees
- Builds strength and corrects muscular imbalances in the hips
- Increases flexibility and mobility in the hips
- Perfect for stretching the groin and releasing tension in the lower back and knees

NICK'S TIP: *I like using Lizard a day or so after strength-training sessions to help loosen up my hips, and particularly my hip flexors.*

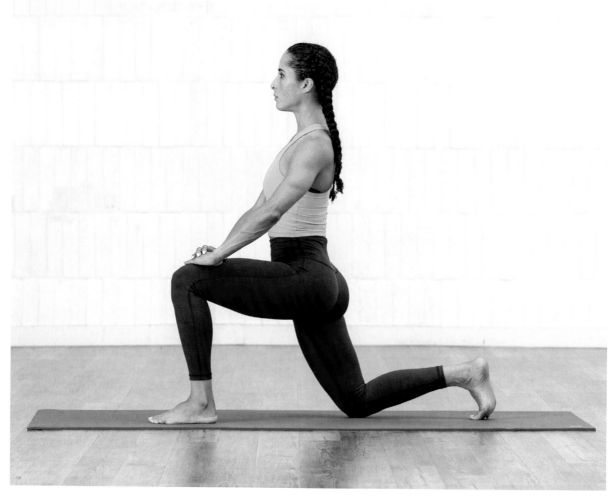

1 From a kneeling, low-lunge position, widen your stance by moving your front foot forward and toward the outside a few inches. Your knee should stay above or slightly past the ankle.

BUILD STRENGTH IN END RANGE: *To build active mobility in your hips, squeeze the glute of the rear leg to deepen the stretch in the corresponding hip flexor.*

BRIAN'S HINT: *You should be able to take a full breath and feel your pelvic floor expanding with the inhale. If you don't, you probably need to rest your hands on a block or come up to your fingertips to keep your torso in a more upright position.*

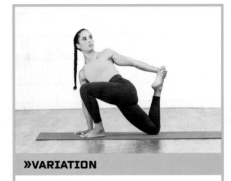

»VARIATION

REACHBACK

For: deeper hip flexor stretch and added quadriceps stretch

Use your hand to grab the corresponding foot or ankle of the back leg and pull the foot toward your outer hip. Use a strap if you need more assistance. Keep your back flat and abs slightly engaged. You can also rest your shin against the wall or on a couch for a hands-free (but still intense) modification.

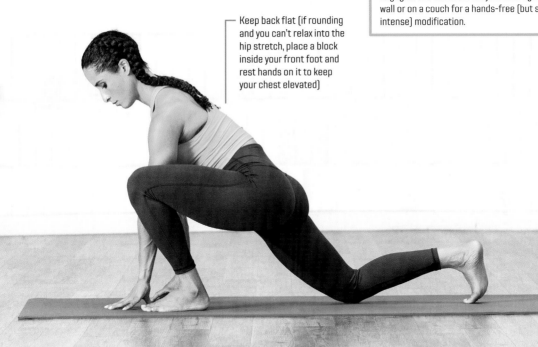

Keep back flat (if rounding and you can't relax into the hip stretch, place a block inside your front foot and rest hands on it to keep your chest elevated)

2 Allow your hips to sink forward and down until you feel an adequate stretch through the hips, making sure you keep your back flat. Rest your fingertips or hands on the ground. If you notice your back rounding, place your hands on a pair of blocks. Inhale to lengthen the front of your torso and lift your spine. Exhale to sink deeper into the hip stretch, bringing your hips further forward and closer to the ground. If you have a great deal of flexibility, you may work toward releasing your forearms to the ground, but only if your back stays flat and your hips stay level. (The focus is on the hip stretch—don't worry about getting your forearms down.)

MOUNTAIN

- Brings awareness to breath and body and improves focus
- Corrects posture
- Perfect for any warm-up or to just check in with your body and see what needs work that day

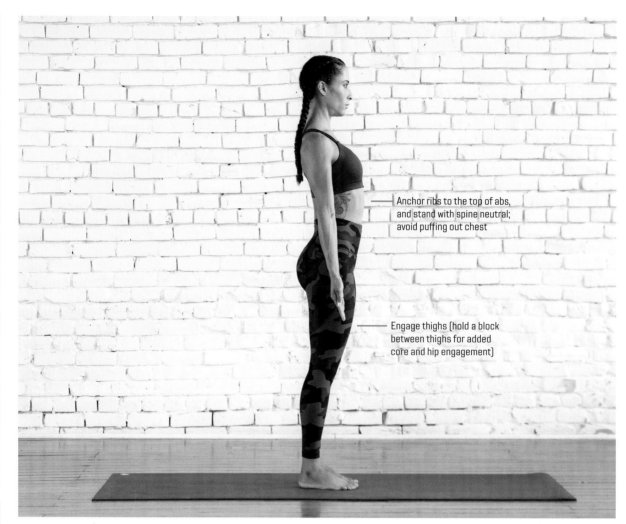

Anchor ribs to the top of abs, and stand with spine neutral; avoid puffing out chest

Engage thighs (hold a block between thighs for added core and hip engagement)

1 Stand with your big toes touching and your heels about 1 inch (2.5cm) apart, insides of your feet parallel to one another and toes facing forward. (If this is uncomfortable, you can stand with your feet at hip width.) Stand with a neutral spine, but keep in mind that your spine has a natural curve to it. When viewed from the side, the lumbar spine (lower back) has a concave (inward) curvature, the thoracic spine (middle back) has a convex (outward) curvature, and the cervical spine (neck) has another concave curvature. Your waist, when at a neutral position, should face just slightly downward.

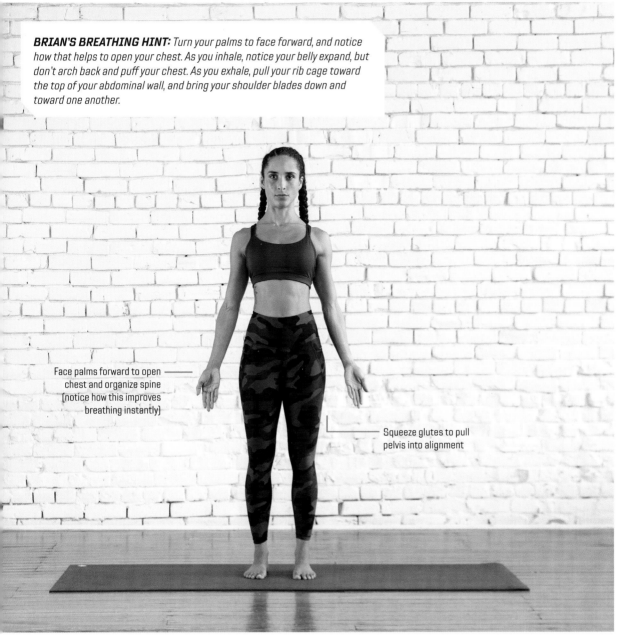

BRIAN'S BREATHING HINT: *Turn your palms to face forward, and notice how that helps to open your chest. As you inhale, notice your belly expand, but don't arch back and puff your chest. As you exhale, pull your rib cage toward the top of your abdominal wall, and bring your shoulder blades down and toward one another.*

Face palms forward to open chest and organize spine (notice how this improves breathing instantly)

Squeeze glutes to pull pelvis into alignment

2 Press down through your heels, balls of the feet, and all five toes to evenly distribute your body weight. (Don't lean forward into your toes. To correct this, lean your hips back slightly. You'll feel your core become more active as you do this.) Slightly flex your knees and squeeze your glutes to reach your tailbone down and guide your pelvis into neutral alignment. Keeping the spine neutral, lift your sternum and press the crown of your head toward the ceiling, chin relaxing toward your throat. Hold your arms at your sides, palms facing forward, shoulder blades lightly pulling down and back. Inhale to expand your chest. Keep your shoulders still as you breathe; avoid lifting them with the inhale. Exhale to empty your lungs and draw your navel to your spine.

PIGEON

- Prevents injury in the hips, knees, and spine
- Builds strength and corrects muscular imbalances in the hips
- Increases flexibility and mobility in the hips
- One of the best overall postures for hip mobility

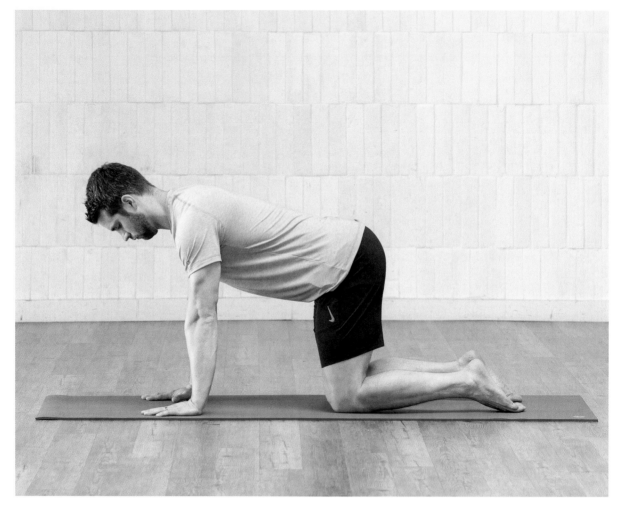

1 Start in a tabletop position with your hips stacked over your knees and your shoulders stacked over your hands. Untuck your toes.

BUILD STRENGTH IN END RANGE: *To build active hip mobility, squeeze the glute of the extended leg, hug your hips toward one another, and shift your weight to your hips. Think of the muscles you would use to lift your leg while in this position—this will help you build active mobility even while you are deep into this pose.*

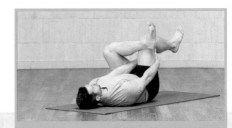

»VARIATION

RECLINED FIGURE 4
For: knee issues or limited hip mobility

Lie on your back, cross one ankle over the opposite thigh (just below the knee), and then grab the back of the noncrossed leg with both hands. Externally rotate the hip of the crossed leg until you feel a stretch in your outer thigh and outer hip. Relax your head and neck as much as you are able. (To increase the effectiveness of the pose, press the foot of your noncrossed leg against a wall.)

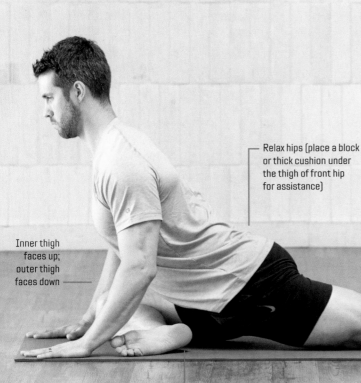

Relax hips (place a block or thick cushion under the thigh of front hip for assistance)

Inner thigh faces up; outer thigh faces down

If you have any knee discomfort, bend knee more to bring heel closer to groin

Keep back leg straight with the tops of thighs and shins facing straight down

2 Slide one knee up toward your hand on the same side, and bring that foot across your body to rest between your opposite hand and knee. (If you're less flexible, bend your knee more; if you're more flexible, work toward a 90-degree bend in your knee.) Externally rotate your hip so your knee is pointed outward, inner thigh facing up, and outer thigh facing down. Extend the toes of your back foot as far back as possible, releasing your hips toward the floor as you do so. Rest your hands in front of the bent leg, and, if necessary, shift your body weight into your hands to help square the hips forward. (With practice and increased flexibility, work toward shifting most or all of your weight to your hips.) Inhale to lengthen your torso forward and up. Exhale to sink your hips deeper.

PYRAMID

- Prevents injury in the spine and hips
- Builds strength and corrects muscular imbalances in the hips and core
- Increases flexibility and mobility in the hips and hamstrings
- Perfect for building strength in spinal flexion

NICK'S TIP: *Endurance athletes have such tight hamstrings, and Pyramid is great for correcting that. I know that sports science tells us to avoid passive stretching before intense exercise, but I have found a nice, long pyramid hold before a run extremely beneficial. This makes sure my calves and hamstrings stay loose and don't cramp up during the run.*

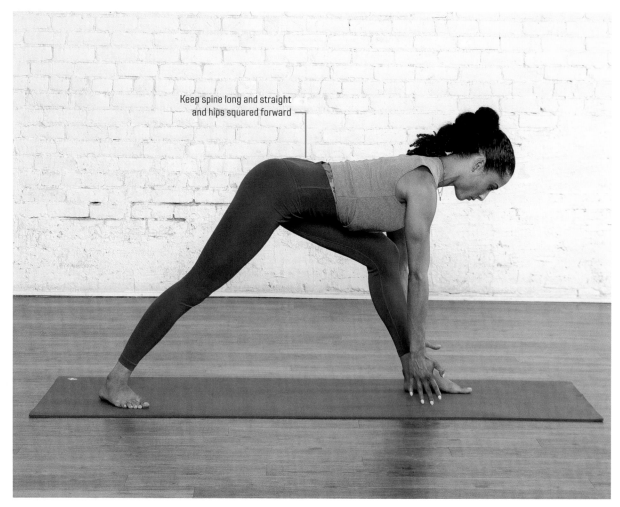

Keep spine long and straight and hips squared forward

1 Start in a shallow lunge position with your back foot turned out to about 45 degrees. Keeping your back flat, lean forward over your front thigh and place your hands on either side of your foot. (You could rest your hands on a pair of blocks.) Pull your chest forward and up to lengthen the front of your torso and lengthen your spine.

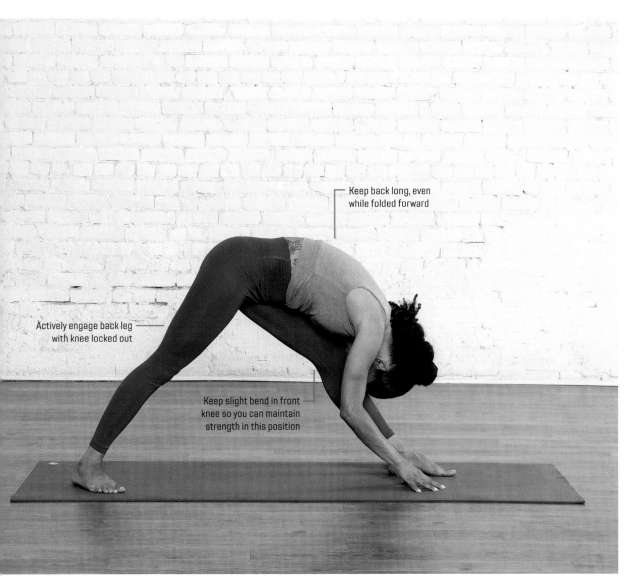

Keep back long, even while folded forward

Actively engage back leg with knee locked out

Keep slight bend in front knee so you can maintain strength in this position

2 Flex your quadriceps, and straighten your front leg until you feel a stretch in your hamstrings. Inhale to pull your chest forward and lift your torso. Exhale to reduce the bend in your front knee and work deeper into the stretch.

RECLINED STRAP STRETCHES

- Prevents injury in the spine, hips, knees, and ankles
- Builds strength and corrects muscular imbalances in the hips and ankles
- Increases flexibility and mobility in the hips
- Perfect restorative stretches for releasing tension in all lower-body joints and lower back, speeding up recovery of the hip and thigh muscles, and increasing overall lower-body flexibility

DEAN'S TIP: *If any of these stretches are difficult, bend your knees. You can also lengthen your grip on the strap or use a door frame to rest your leg directly against a wall (instead of having to hold it with a strap).*

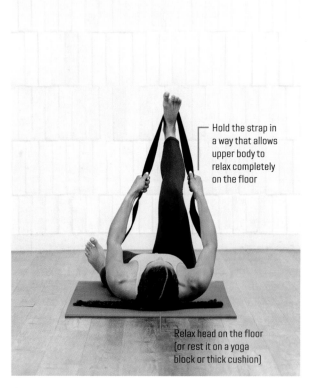

Hold the strap in a way that allows upper body to relax completely on the floor

Relax head on the floor (or rest it on a yoga block or thick cushion)

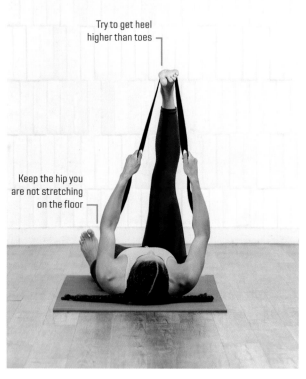

Try to get heel higher than toes

Keep the hip you are not stretching on the floor

1 Lie on your back. Position a strap on the arch of one foot, and hold the ends of the strap with both hands. Rest your other leg on the floor. Relax your shoulders and back on the floor. Slightly tuck your chin to keep your neck and spine neutral. Do any of the next three stretches for the hamstrings, adductors, or abductors. For each, inhale to lengthen the extended leg. Exhale to stretch deeper.

2 **Hamstring Strap Stretch:** Keeping the extended leg flat on the floor, straighten your other leg as much as possible while keeping your back flat. Reach the toes of your lifted foot toward your shin and press your heel up to stretch your calf. (Depending on your hamstring flexibility, you may or may not need to bend your knee.) Squeeze your quadriceps to help lengthen your hamstrings and accentuate the stretch.

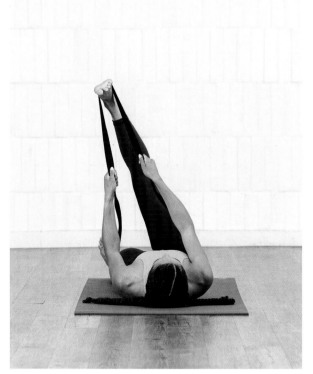

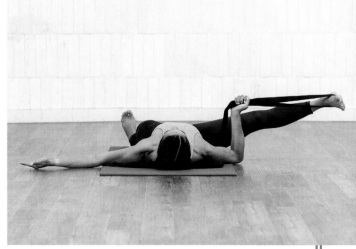

3 **Abductor Strap Stretch:** Keeping the extended leg flat on the floor, bring the leg you are stretching in the strap just a few inches toward the opposite inner thigh, coming across your body, until you feel a stretch in the outer thigh and hip. Keep both hips flat on the floor.

4 **Adductor Strap Stretch:** Keeping the extended leg flat on the floor, bring the leg you are stretching in the strap toward the outside until you feel a sufficient stretch in your inner thigh. Keep the hip of the nonstretching leg in contact with the floor. Slightly bend your knee to help focus the stretch on the inner thigh. (You shouldn't feel pulling close to the knee.)

RECLINED TWIST

- Prevents injury in the spine and shoulders
- Builds strength and corrects muscular imbalances in the core, spine, and hips
- Increases flexibility and mobility in the spine, hips, and shoulders
- Perfect for opening the lumbar spine and releasing lower-back stiffness, as well as preparing the back for exercise

FRANCHESKA'S TIP: *My favorite way to incorporate this pose into my routine is as a cooldown with breath work. Spending time in this active spinal rotation helps relieve tons of tension throughout the entire spine.*

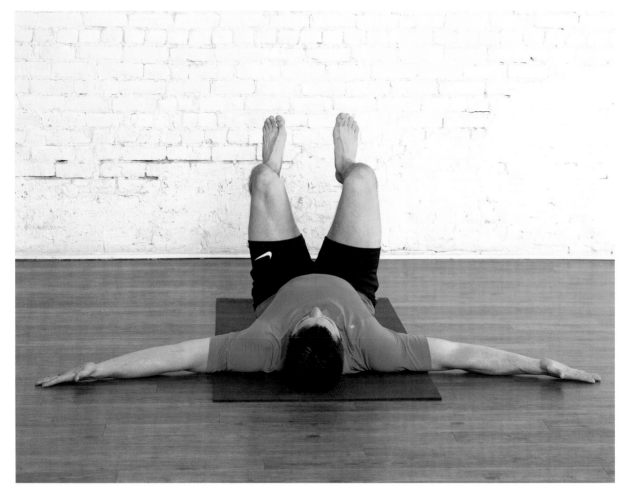

1 Lie on your back with your knees directly over your hips. Extend your arms directly out to the sides with palms facing the ceiling.

BUILD STRENGTH IN END RANGE: *Actively press the arm and shoulder (opposite your twist) into the ground. Use the opposite hand to press your stacked knees into the floor to build more active mobility in your hips and spine.*

BRIAN'S BREATHING HINT: *Inhale as deep as you can to help achieve greater range of motion in the twist. The exhale helps you go deeper, but the inhale helps you own that greater range of motion.*

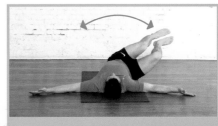

»VARIATION

REPS

For: added core strengthening

While keeping your shoulders planted, inhale to lower your legs sideways; hover just off the ground. Then exhale to squeeze your abs and bring your legs back to the middle. Repeat on the other side, and keep alternating back and forth, or for 5 to 10 reps per side.

If you can't get knees to the ground while keeping shoulders down, place a block or cushion under the knees

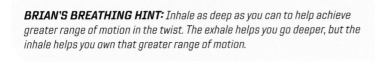

Keep shoulder down while twisting (if you can't yet, it will come with practice)

2 Lower your legs to one side, keeping the legs stacked and doing your best to keep your shoulders on the ground. (If they come up a little, that's okay.) Place your hand on your stacked knees. Draw in your chest to keep your spine neutral and to help deepen the stretch in your back. Press the crown of your head away from your shoulders. Inhale to maintain your position. Exhale to squeeze your core and deepen the twist.

RUNNER'S LUNGE TWIST

- Prevents injury in the spine, shoulders, hips, and ankles
- Builds strength and corrects muscular imbalances in the shoulders, upper back, core, hips, and ankles
- Increases flexibility and mobility in the shoulders, spine, and hips
- Perfect full-body posture for warming up, building lower-body strength and mobility, improving thoracic and overall spinal mobility, increasing core strength, and improving balance

FRANCHESKA'S TIP: *Who said yoga was easy? Maintaining full-body engagement in this twisting lunge is one of my favorite ways to strengthen and mobilize the hips and spine. Actively try to lengthen through your spine as you hold this pose.*

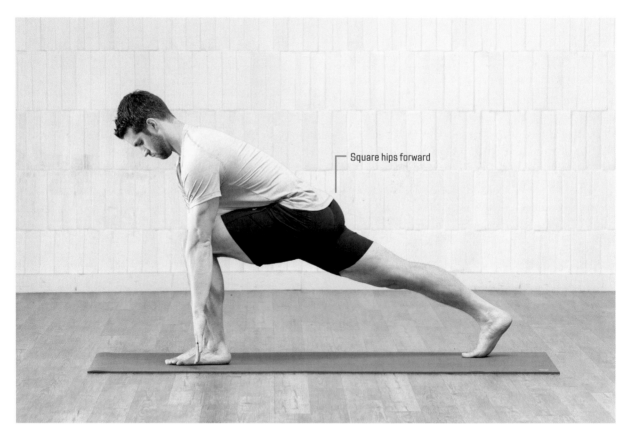

Square hips forward

1 Start in Runner's Lunge with your front knee over your ankle and your back knee as close to locked out as possible, fingertips resting on the floor. (Use a block inside your front foot if you notice your back rounding with your fingers on the floor.)

BUILD STRENGTH IN END RANGE: *Use the hand that's resting on the floor (or block) as a guide for balance rather than putting your body weight into it. The less weight you rest in your hand to assist with balance, the more challenging you make this for your lower body. Squeeze your feet toward your midline.*

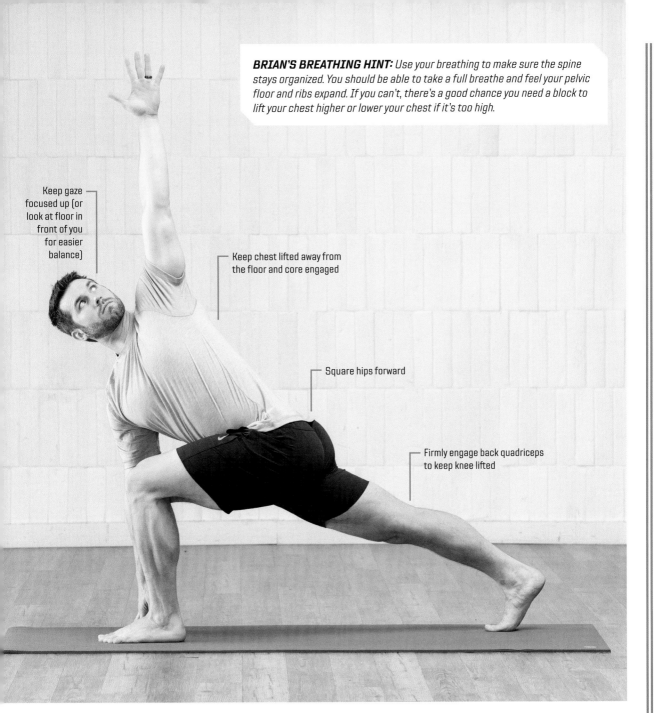

BRIAN'S BREATHING HINT: *Use your breathing to make sure the spine stays organized. You should be able to take a full breathe and feel your pelvic floor and ribs expand. If you can't, there's a good chance you need a block to lift your chest higher or lower your chest if it's too high.*

Keep gaze focused up (or look at floor in front of you for easier balance)

Keep chest lifted away from the floor and core engaged

Square hips forward

Firmly engage back quadriceps to keep knee lifted

2 Inhale to lengthen your chest forward and press the crown of your head away from your hips. Keeping your hips and lower body squared, rotate your torso toward your bent leg and extend that arm up toward the ceiling. Lightly rest (or don't rest at all) your other hand on the floor to make this more challenging.

Once you feel balanced, turn your head to look up at your extended arm. Maintain length in your neck, chin tucked in toward your throat. Do not allow the hip of your extended leg to dip toward the floor. Inhale to lengthen the torso and expand in all directions. Exhale to deepen the rotation and reach the arm further back and higher.

SEATED TWIST

- Prevents injury in the spine, shoulders, hips, and knees
- Builds strength and corrects muscular imbalances in the spine, hips, and core
- Increases flexibility and mobility in the spine and hips
- Perfect for increasing spinal mobility while building core and hip strength

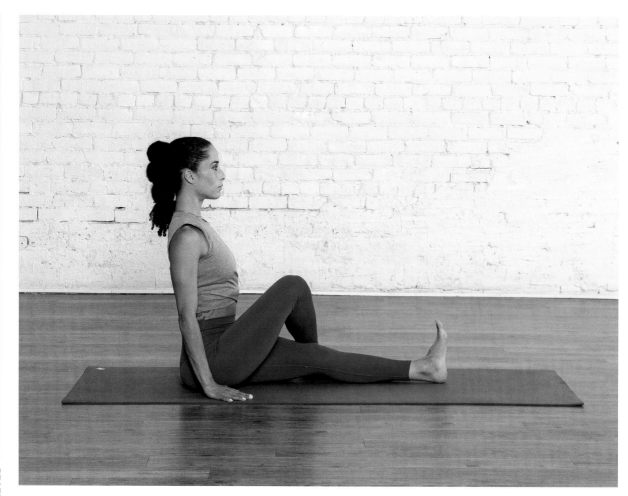

1 From a strong, upright seated position, extend one leg straight out in front of you. Cross your other leg over, planting that foot outside the opposite knee.

BUILD STRENGTH IN END RANGE: *To build active mobility in your hips and spine, hover your elbow above your knee and use your core strength to actively hold your torso upright in the twist.*

2 Bring the opposite hand around your bent knee, and lightly plant your other hand behind the hip of your crossed leg. Sit as upright as you can, actively engaging your pelvic floor and core by rooting down through your hips and lifting the ribs away from the floor. Avoid cranking your elbow into your knee to force the twist. Inhale to get taller and add length to your spine. Exhale to work deeper, with control, into the twist.

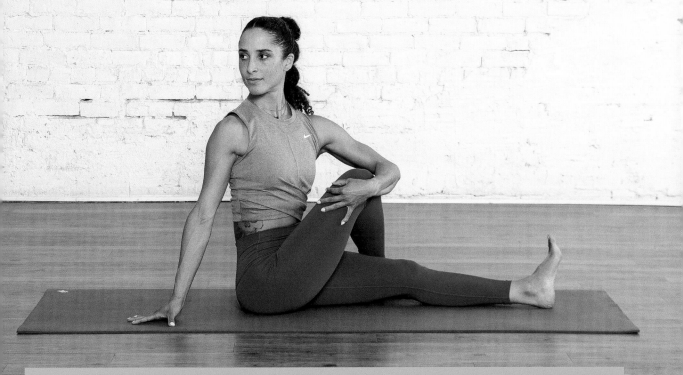

» VARIATIONS

KNEE TO CHEST
For: a more relaxed or beginner-friendly version

Use both hands to lightly hug your knee in toward your chest. Continue to use your hips and core to hold yourself upright. You should feel a stretch through your outer thigh and hip.

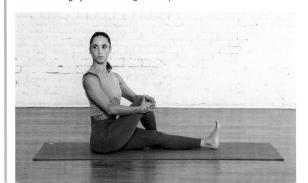

ELBOW TO KNEE
For: a more active, deeper version

Bring your elbow to the outside of the opposite knee. Make sure you have the core strength and active mobility to be able to *mostly* reach this position without relying on the elbow.

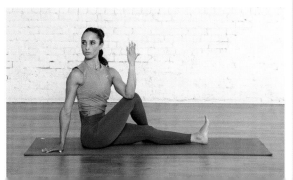

SIDE ANGLE

- Prevents injury in the spine, shoulders, hips, and ankles
- Builds strength and corrects muscular imbalances in the shoulders, upper back, core, hips, and ankles
- Increases flexibility and mobility in the upper back, shoulders, hips, and ankles
- Perfect for improving balance while working the entire lower body and core

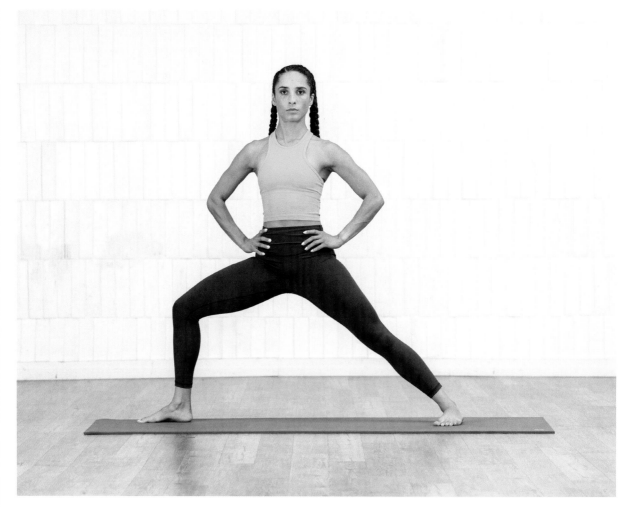

1 Start in Warrior 2 (p. 168) with your feet 4 to 5 feet (1.25–1.5m) apart, your feet perpendicular, and your forward knee bent directly over your ankle.

BUILD STRENGTH IN END RANGE: *To build active lower-body mobility, hug your legs toward one another, squeeze your glutes and quadriceps, and press into the outer edges of your feet. To build active core, spine, and shoulder mobility, press your arms in opposite directions and avoid resting your arms or hands on any surface or body part.*

BRIAN'S BREATHING HINT: *As you inhale, maintain your height and keep an upright torso. You should be able to notice the air expanding in your lower back and ribs. If you can't, make sure you are keeping your core lifted and not allowing your chest to slump downward. As you exhale, sink deeper into the lunge, maintaining the feeling of "lift" in your chest as you do so.*

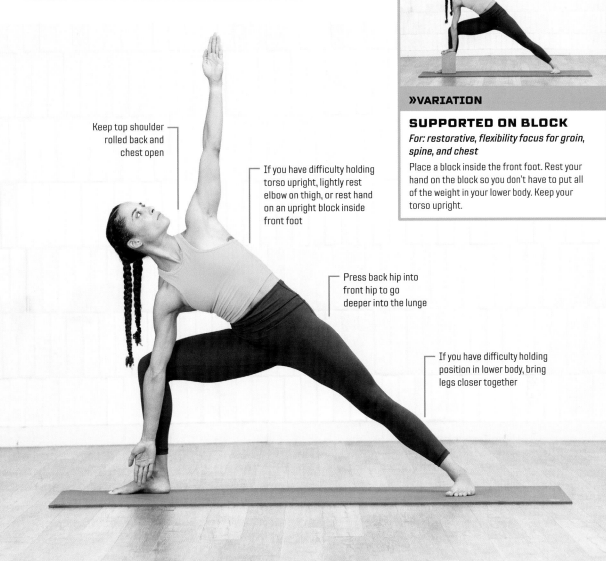

»VARIATION

SUPPORTED ON BLOCK

For: restorative, flexibility focus for groin, spine, and chest

Place a block inside the front foot. Rest your hand on the block so you don't have to put all of the weight in your lower body. Keep your torso upright.

Keep top shoulder rolled back and chest open

If you have difficulty holding torso upright, lightly rest elbow on thigh, or rest hand on an upright block inside front foot

Press back hip into front hip to go deeper into the lunge

If you have difficulty holding position in lower body, bring legs closer together

2 Lean your torso toward the bent leg to form a line from your extended leg through the torso to your head. Stretch your arms vertically from the floor to the ceiling, palms facing forward, so that your lower elbow grazes your inner thigh. If your hand touches the ground, don't shift your body weight into it. Press your hands in opposite directions as you peel back your top shoulder and open your chest toward the sky. Look up at your left hand. Press the crown of your head away from the shoulders. Keep your hips centered between your feet, not allowing your hips to poke out behind you. Inhale to lengthen the torso. Exhale to deepen the twist.

SIDE PLANK

- Prevents injury in the spine, shoulders, hips, knees, and ankles
- Builds strength and corrects muscular imbalances in the shoulders, upper back, core, spine, hips, and lower body
- Increases flexibility and mobility in the hips and spine
- Perfect for full-body strength and muscle activation, targeting the hips, core, and shoulders Great for any warm-up or standalone workout

FRANCHESKA'S TIP: *Here's another training gap: lateral stability. It's essential for injury prevention and athletic performance! Take note of how much stronger you feel after training for lateral stability.*

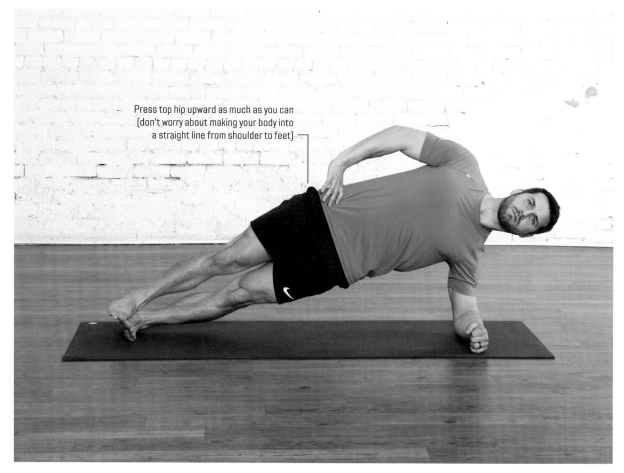

Press top hip upward as much as you can (don't worry about making your body into a straight line from shoulder to feet)

1 Lie on your side and place your top hand on your hip. Resting on your forearm, use your hips and core strength to lift your body, keeping your hips and shoulders vertically stacked. If you need strength or balance support, bend and plant your knees instead of your feet. Make sure your hips aren't sticking out behind you.

»VARIATION

LIFTED LEG

For: building more strength

Lift the top leg away from the planted leg, squeezing your outer hip upward. Avoid turning your hips out; make sure your toes face directly sideways. Continue to drive your hips upward.

To make easier, unstack legs and stagger feet on the floor, or bend and stack knees, and rest knees and ankles on ground

Feel your weight in upper back, not front of shoulder

BUILD STRENGTH IN END RANGE: *To maximize active core mobility, continue to drive your hips upward. In the advanced variation (Lifted Leg), pull the outside of your lifted foot straight upward as high as possible while keeping your hips squared forward.*

2 Drive your hips up as high as possible. Extend your nonplanted arm straight upward, forming a straight line from your planted elbow to your extended hand. Pull the crown of your head away from your chest, and rotate your head to look up at your hand. Inhale to lengthen your torso. Exhale as you reach your arm and hips higher.

STANDING BACKBEND

- Prevents injury in the spine, shoulders, and hips
- Builds strength and corrects muscular imbalances in the shoulders, upper back, spine, core, and hips
- Increases flexibility and mobility in the spine and shoulders
- Perfect for warming up the core and upper body for exercise

FRANCHESKA'S TIP: *Instead of focusing on how deep you can go in this backbend, prioritize lengthening through your spine and keeping your abdomen and pelvic floor engaged. If you feel limited here, try looking up toward your brow for more range of motion.*

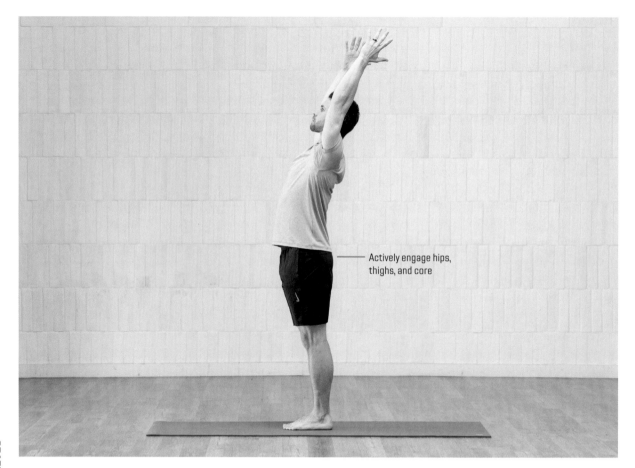

Actively engage hips, thighs, and core

1 Stand in an active Mountain (p. 136) with your big toes touching and your heels about 1 inch (2.5cm) apart. Keep your thighs, hips, and core slightly engaged. (If this is uncomfortable, plant your feet at hip width, and consider holding a block between your legs.) Lift your arms overhead, palms facing each other.

BUILD STRENGTH IN END RANGE: *To build active mobility in your upper back and shoulders, squeeze your arms as far back as possible. To build active mobility in your spine, keep your core firmly engaged as you go deeper into the backbend.*

BRIAN'S BREATHING HINT: *If you notice your inhale is restricted in your throat, make sure you have proper neck positioning. You should still be feeling your ribs expand in the front, and the focus should be on opening your chest, not your neck. Lastly, acknowledge that this is not a position where you'll be able to breathe normally, and that's okay.*

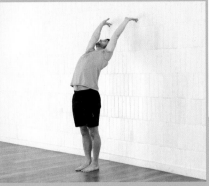

»VARIATION

ON WALL
For: focus on flexibility

Stand with your back 1 to 2 feet (30.5cm–0.5m) away from a wall. Reach your hands up and back and use the wall to support your backbend. Avoid pinching in your lower back; keep the focus on arching from the midback and up.

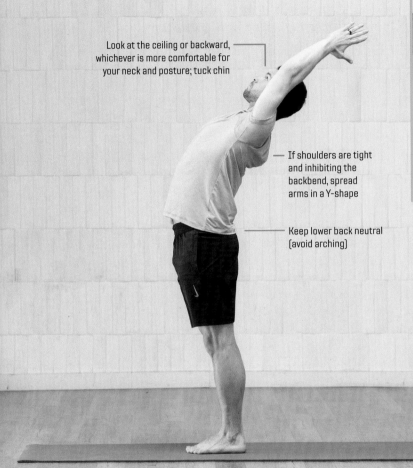

Look at the ceiling or backward, whichever is more comfortable for your neck and posture; tuck chin

If shoulders are tight and inhibiting the backbend, spread arms in a Y-shape

Keep lower back neutral (avoid arching)

2 Press your palms together, and lock out your arms. Keeping length in your neck, look upward and squeeze your arms back as far as possible, coming into a strong backbend. Bend from your midback and up; don't allow your lower back to arch. Instead of "falling" backward, press your fingers up and then squeeze back, maintaining strength in the backbend. Keep your core tight and hips and thighs firmly engaged. Bend back only as far as it feels comfortable while your core remains engaged. Do not allow the back of your neck to collapse. As you inhale, lengthen the spine and grow taller. As you exhale, increase the degree of the backbend and reach further back. (There is a constant push and pull of arching further back and getting taller during this pose.)

STANDING BOW

- Prevents injury in the spine, hips, ankles, knees, and shoulders
- Builds strength and corrects muscular imbalances in the shoulders, upper back, core, hips, and ankles
- Increases flexibility and mobility in the shoulders, hips, and ankles
- Perfect for targeting hip flexor mobility, increasing overall hip mobility, and improving balance

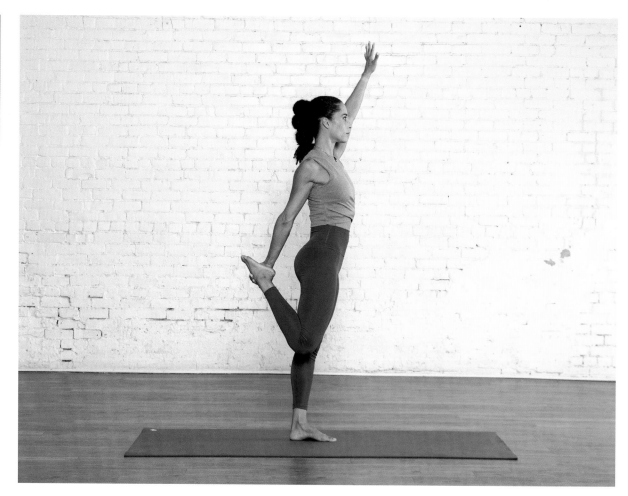

1 Balance on one leg. Bend the knee of your lifted leg back, and bring that heel toward your glutes. Use the corresponding hand to grab the inside of your foot, keeping your shoulder open as you do so. Press down firmly through the standing leg, and extend the corresponding arm straight up, biceps next to your ear.

BUILD STRENGTH IN END RANGE: *To build active hip mobility, in your lifted leg, squeeze your glute and actively press your foot into your hand.*

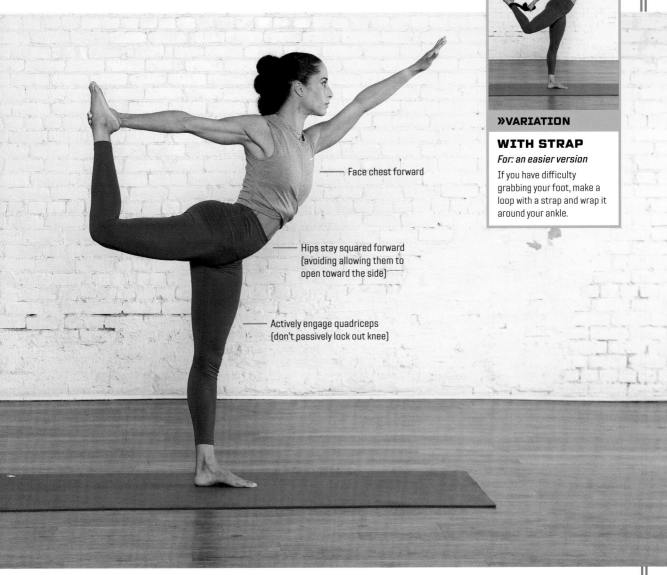

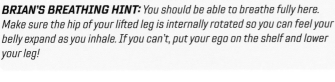

»VARIATION

WITH STRAP

For: an easier version

If you have difficulty grabbing your foot, make a loop with a strap and wrap it around your ankle.

— Face chest forward

— Hips stay squared forward (avoiding allowing them to open toward the side)

— Actively engage quadriceps (don't passively lock out knee)

2 Inhale and lengthen your body to get as tall as possible. Then exhale as you press your lifted foot into your hand and hinge at the hips to bring your torso forward and down while your lifted leg comes up and back. Keep your hips squared forward; avoid turning the hips sideways in an effort to lift your leg higher. Keep your core engaged and reach your tailbone back to maintain length in your lower back. Inhale to lengthen your body and maintain proper alignment. Exhale to work deeper into the hip opening and bring your chest further forward and down.

STANDING SIDEBEND

- Prevents injury in the spine, shoulders, and hips
- Builds strength and corrects muscular imbalances in the shoulders, upper back, core, and hips
- Increases flexibility and mobility in the shoulders, hips, and spine
- Perfect for increasing side-flexion spinal strength and mobility

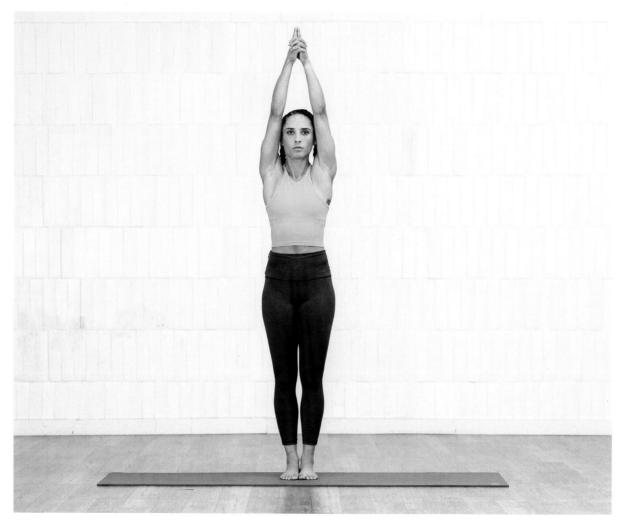

1 Stand in an active Mountain (p. 136) with your big toes touching and your heels about 1 inch (2.5cm) apart. Keep your thighs, hips, and core slightly engaged. (If this is uncomfortable, plant your feet at hip width, and consider holding a block between your legs.) Reach your arms overhead, press your palms together, and interlace your fingers, pointing the index fingers up. Rotate your arms inward so your biceps face your ears. Lock your arms in this position.

BRIAN'S BREATHING HINT: *As you inhale, think about expanding your rib cage in whichever side you are trying to stretch. (If you're leaning toward the right, focus on expanding into your left rib cage.) Take a 1 to 2 second pause between the inhale and exhale to give your muscles a chance to open.*

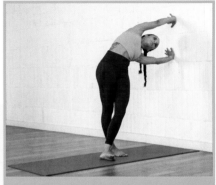

»VARIATION

ON WALL

For: a more relaxed flexibility focus

Stand with your side to a wall, feet planted a few feet from the wall. Reach up and over your head, bending toward the wall, and place your hands at shoulder height (as if you were going to do a cartwheel on the wall). Lean into the wall as you stretch your side. If your side feels restricted, cross the foot that's closer to the wall over the opposite foot.

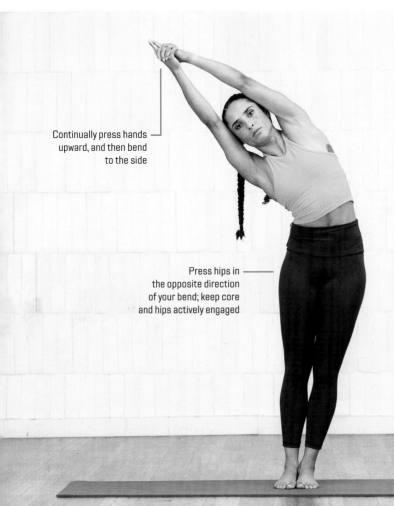

Continually press hands upward, and then bend to the side

Press hips in the opposite direction of your bend; keep core and hips actively engaged

BUILD STRENGTH IN END RANGE: *For active upper-body mobility, maintain intense core and thigh engagement (knees locked out, quadriceps engaged) and continue to squeeze your arms backward without arching your back. For an even greater upper-body challenge, press your palms together instead of interlacing your fingers.*

2 Reach up as high as you can, and then lean toward one side with your upper body, pressing your hips in the opposite direction. Squeeze your quadriceps to keep your legs straight and hips active. Use your inhale to get taller and reset your posture. Exhale to go deeper into the bend while maintaining strength through your core, hips, and spine.

THREAD THE NEEDLE

- Prevents injury in the spine and shoulders
- Builds strength and corrects muscular imbalances in the shoulders, upper back, and spine
- Increases flexibility and mobility in the shoulders and spine
- Great stretch for the scapular stabilizers and for improving passive thoracic mobility

NICK'S TIP: *I find this posture incredibly useful one to two days after a big back or chest workout. Strength training is accompanied by mobility restriction, so I'll use this pose to help get out in front of that.*

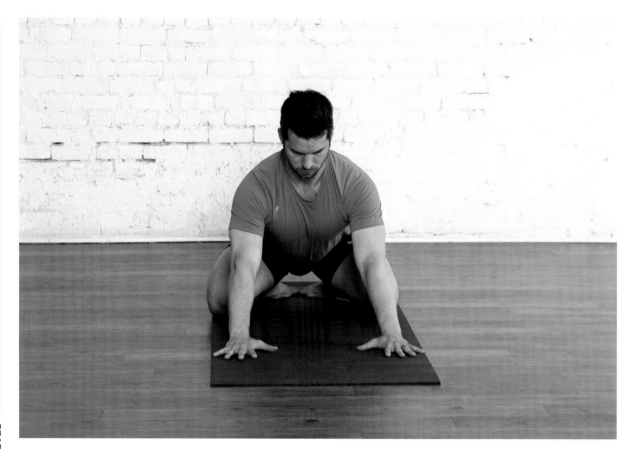

1 Start in Child's Pose (p. 116) with your knees wider than your shoulders, big toes touching, and hips shifted back toward your heels. Keep your arms and torso long.

BUILD STRENGTH IN END RANGE: *To intensify the stretch, press the back of the arm and shoulder that you are stretching into the ground, and lightly "pull" it back across your body (without actually moving it).*

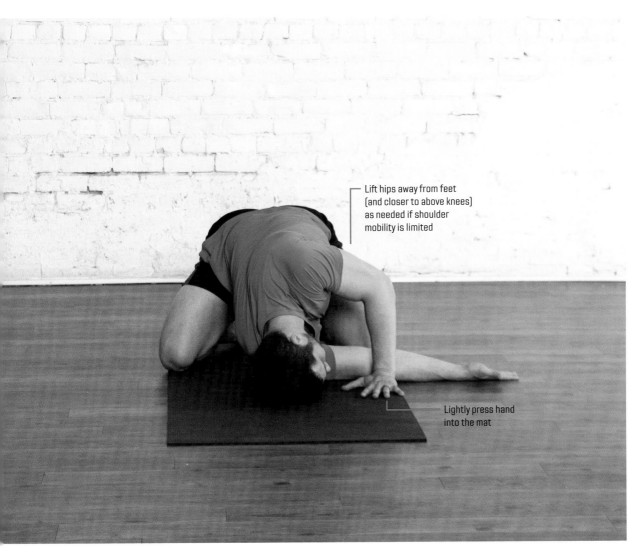

Lift hips away from feet (and closer to above knees) as needed if shoulder mobility is limited

Lightly press hand into the mat

2 Slide one arm under the other, between your hand and knee, palm facing up. Look toward your threaded hand, and relax your head onto the mat. Focus on stretching your threaded shoulder blade and twisting through your midback. Keep your glutes as close to your heels as you comfortably can, and avoid twisting your lower back. Inhale to expand your back and shoulders. Exhale to deepen the shoulder stretch, pressing your arm into the floor.

TREE

- Prevents injury in the spine, shoulders, hips, and ankles
- Builds strength and corrects muscular imbalances in the shoulders, upper back, core, hips, and ankles
- Increases flexibility and mobility in the shoulders and hips
- Perfect for developing balance and building lower-body joint stability while strengthening your hips

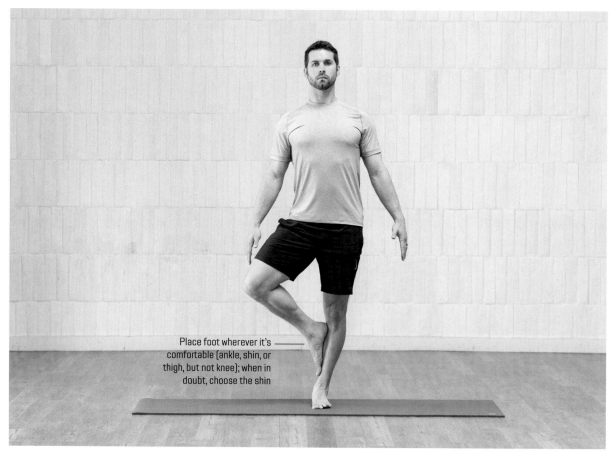

Place foot wherever it's comfortable (ankle, shin, or thigh, but not knee); when in doubt, choose the shin

1 Starting from a standing position, shift your body weight into one foot. Press the sole of the opposite foot into the shin or thigh of the standing leg. Keeping your hips squared forward, externally rotate the hip and squeeze the glutes so the knee faces the side. Squeeze your lifted foot upward to activate your hamstrings and further strengthen the hips.

BUILD STRENGTH IN END RANGE: *To build active knee-flexion mobility, maintain active glute engagement in both hips, and hug the heel of the nonstanding leg up toward your groin. To build active shoulder and upper-back mobility, squeeze your arms backward as much as possible.*

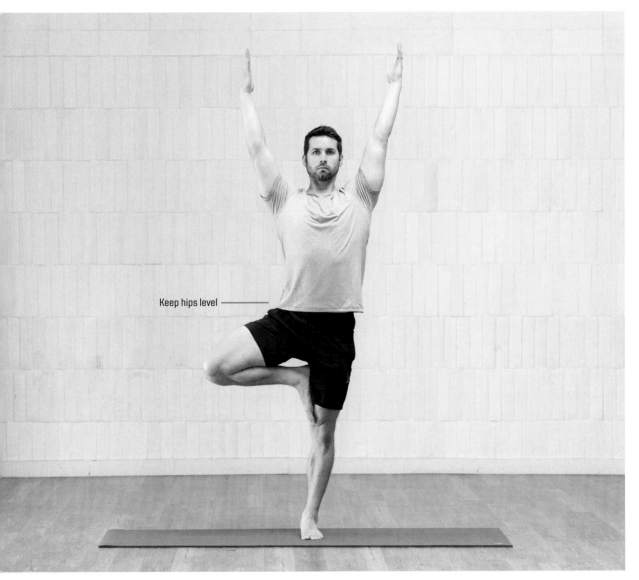

Keep hips level ⎯⎯⎯⎯⎯⎯

2 Lengthen your ribs away from your hips, and extend your arms in a V-shape overhead. To intensify the hip engagement, shift your foot up on your leg, if able. Press down firmly with your planted foot, and grab the ground with your toes to keep the balancing leg active for the duration of the posture. Inhale to lengthen the torso. Exhale to increase engagement of core, thighs, and hips.

TRIANGLE

- Prevents injury in the knees, hips, back, and shoulders
- Builds strength and corrects muscular imbalances in the shoulders, upper back, core, and hips
- Increases flexibility and mobility in the shoulders and hips
- Perfect unilateral posture for increasing inner-thigh mobility

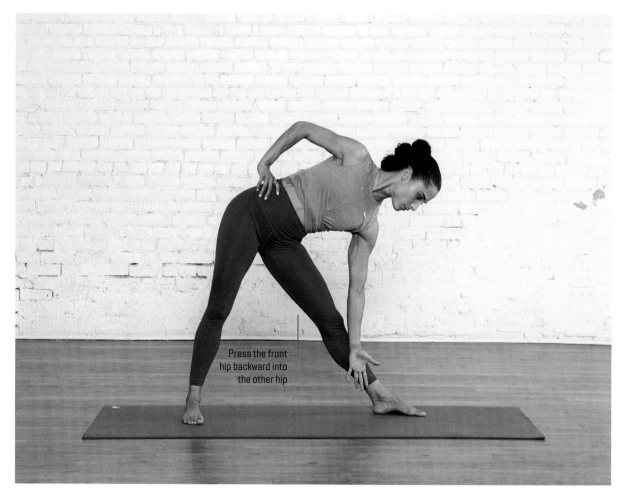

Press the front hip backward into the other hip

1 Stand with your feet slightly wider than shoulder width apart, front foot facing the top of the mat, and back toes turned slightly in. Reach down to extend one arm to the inside of your front foot, maintaining a straight line through your core (not rounding through your sides). Keep a slight bend to your front knee, bending it more if you are less flexible. The back leg should stay locked out with quadriceps firmly engaged.

BUILD STRENGTH IN END RANGE: *Hug your legs toward one another, and lift your hand off the block or ground (so you are not supporting any body weight with your arm) to build more active mobility in your hips and core.*

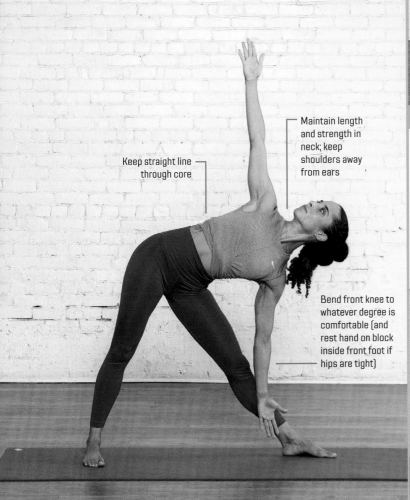

Keep straight line through core

Maintain length and strength in neck; keep shoulders away from ears

Bend front knee to whatever degree is comfortable (and rest hand on block inside front foot if hips are tight)

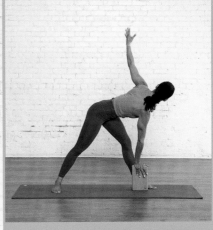

»VARIATION

REVOLVED

For: rotation and spinal mobility

Turn your back foot in slightly more than you would for a standard Triangle. From Triangle, turn to place your raised hand on a block inside your front foot. (If you're very flexible, you can try placing your hand directly on the floor on either side of your foot.) Pull your chest forward to lengthen your spine. Twist open in the direction of your front foot, focusing on using your spine to open into the twist, not turning your hips.

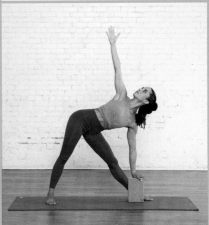

»VARIATION

SUPPORTED ON BLOCK

For: restorative, flexibility focus

Place a block inside your front foot. Rest your hand there to give your lower body and core a bit of a break. Set the block to whatever height enables you to keep your back flat.

2 Extend your other arm upward, palm facing outward, doing your best to form a straight vertical line from hand to hand. Roll your top shoulder back so your torso faces straight out. Inhale to press the top of your head in the same direction your front foot is facing to lengthen your spine, and then slowly look up to face your hand. Exhale to press your front hip toward your back hip and go deeper into the hip stretch and open your torso further into the twist.

WARRIOR 1

- Prevents injury in the spine, hips, ankles, and shoulders
- Builds strength and corrects muscular imbalances in the hips, core, ankles, and shoulders
- Increases flexibility and mobility in the hips, ankles, and shoulders
- Perfect for improving groin and ankle mobility

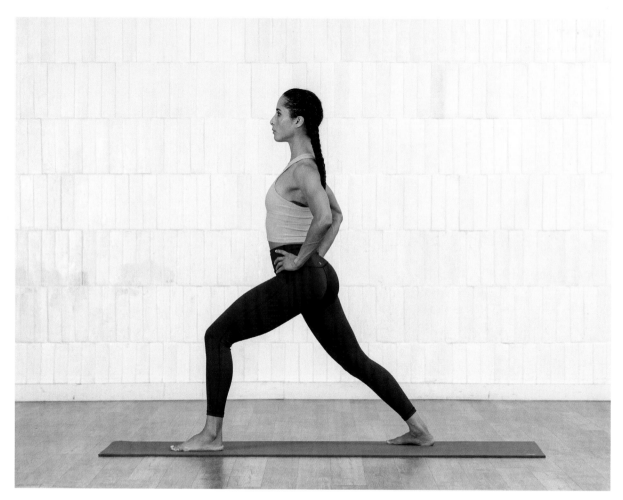

1 Start in a lunge position with your back foot planted about hip width outside your front foot (instead of in a straight line from heel to heel) and pointed out about 45 degrees. Keep your back leg straight, and bend into your front leg until your knee is directly above the ankle, shin perpendicular to the ground. Your lower back should be neutral (not arched), and you should feel a stretch through your groin. Widen your stance if you do not feel a stretch, and bring your feet closer together if your lower back is noticeably arched. Lift your ribs away from your hips to create space in the hips and engage your core.

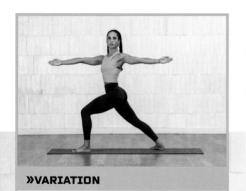

»VARIATION

TWIST

For: spinal mobility and shoulder opening

Keeping your hips squared forward, twist with your upper body in the direction of whichever foot is forward. Extend your arms in opposite directions at shoulder level. You'll feel the muscles in your upper back engage as you hold this. Interlace your fingers behind your neck to isolate the twist in your upper back.

If shoulders are tight and you struggle to get arms overhead without arching back, try goalpost arms instead (bending elbows to 90 degrees and lowering elbows to shoulder level)

Create a long line from extended hip up to the opposing shoulder

Keep back heel and outer edge of foot pressing down, maintaining a strong, lifted arch

BUILD STRENGTH IN END RANGE: *To build active mobility in your adductors and hip flexors, squeeze your legs toward one another. To build active mobility in your upper back, squeeze your arms as far back as possible without arching your back.*

2 Extend your arms overhead and squeeze them as far back as possible, keeping your back flat (no arching or puffing your chest out). Press into the outer edge and heel of your back foot to stretch your ankle, and square your hips forward as much as possible. Inhale to lengthen and get taller. Exhale to sink deeper into the lunge.

WARRIOR 2

- Prevents injury in the spine, knees, hips, ankles, and shoulders
- Builds strength and corrects muscular imbalances in the shoulders, upper back, core, hips, and ankles
- Increases flexibility and mobility in the shoulders, hips, and ankles
- Perfect for actively opening your groin, addressing back stiffness, and correcting anterior pelvic tilt

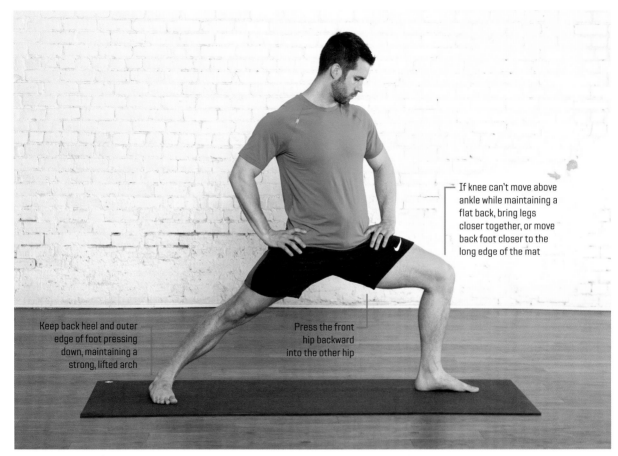

If knee can't move above ankle while maintaining a flat back, bring legs closer together, or move back foot closer to the long edge of the mat

Keep back heel and outer edge of foot pressing down, maintaining a strong, lifted arch

Press the front hip backward into the other hip

1 Start in a wide-legged stance with your feet 4 to 5 feet (1.25–1.5m) apart and toes pointed slightly inward. You should feel light stretching in both sides of the groin. Turn one foot to face straight out and bend the front knee until it is directly over your ankle, keeping hips and shoulders squared to the side (not facing forward). Try to keep your hips level (back hip not higher than the front hip).

BUILD STRENGTH IN END RANGE: *To build inner-thigh mobility, hug your legs toward each other. To build active hip and ankle mobility, squeeze your glutes and quadriceps, and press into the outer edges of your feet.*

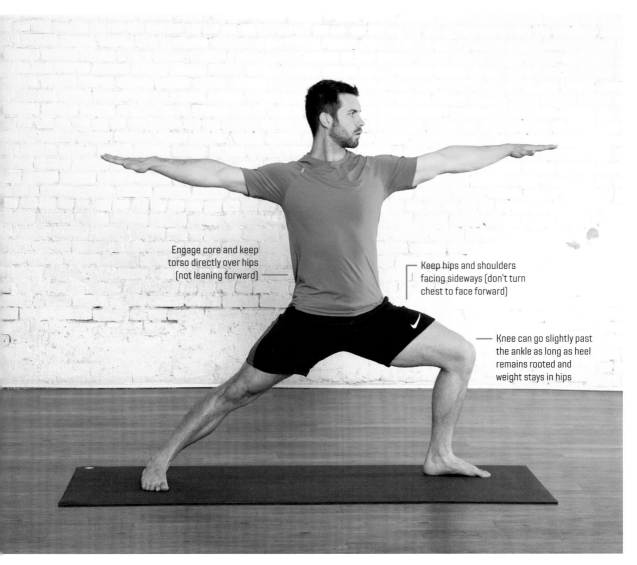

Engage core and keep torso directly over hips (not leaning forward)

Keep hips and shoulders facing sideways (don't turn chest to face forward)

Knee can go slightly past the ankle as long as heel remains rooted and weight stays in hips

2 Keeping your torso over your hips, extend your arms to the sides, palms facing down, and press the fingertips of your opposite hands away from each other. Turn your head and look directly past your front middle finger. Lift your ribs away from your hips to engage your core and create space in the hips. Continue to squeeze your glutes so that your hips remain in proper pelvic alignment with your spine neutral. Inhale to lengthen the spine and grow taller. Exhale to sink deeper into the lunge.

WIDE-LEGGED FORWARD FOLD

- Prevents injury in the spine, hips, ankles, and shoulders
- Builds strength and corrects muscular imbalances in the hips, ankles, core, and shoulders
- Increases flexibility and mobility in the shoulders, hips, and ankles
- Perfect for building active mobility in the inner thighs and hamstrings, while also increasing overall mobility for shoulder extension (when using variation with strap)

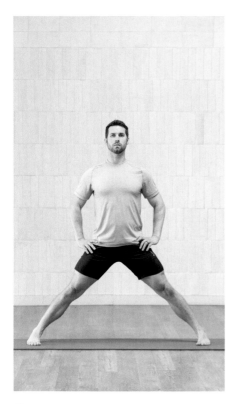

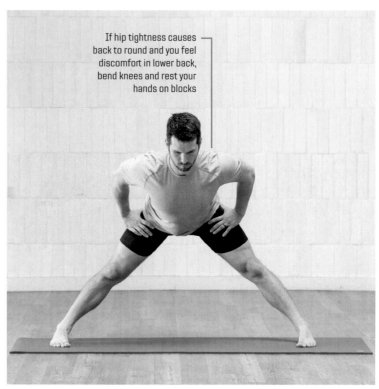

If hip tightness causes back to round and you feel discomfort in lower back, bend knees and rest your hands on blocks

1 Start in a wide-legged stance with your toes turned slightly in. (Your stance should be wide enough that you feel stretching in your groin, but not so wide that you feel uncontrolled.)

2 Press into the outer edges of your feet, squeeze your quadriceps, and hinge at the hips to bring your chest forward and down into a forward fold. Slightly bend your knees, and maintain a firmly engaged core to avoid rounding your back. It helps to think about pressing your lower back down toward your abs and lengthening your inner thighs and hamstrings rather than just trying to get your chest to the floor. Inhale to lengthen your spine and expand your chest. Exhale to work deeper into the forward fold while using your core strength to flex your spine. If your back remains mostly flat (your lower back shouldn't be higher than your hips), move to step 3.

BRIAN'S BREATHING HINT: *Before you fold here, take a full inhale and take a 3-second pause to make sure your hips and spine are in a neutral position, then exhale to squeeze your rib cage to the top of your abdominal muscles. This prepares your spine for a strong forward fold that protects your spine when rounding.*

3 Relax your hands on the floor, but maintain muscle engagement in your quadriceps, hips, and core. (If your hands do not comfortably touch the ground, rest your hands on a block or two.)

BUILD STRENGTH IN END RANGE: *To build active inner-thigh mobility, hug your feet toward one another (as if the mat were sliding apart). To build active core strength, lift your hands off the ground, extend your arms forward, and keep a straight line from your hips to your fingertips.*

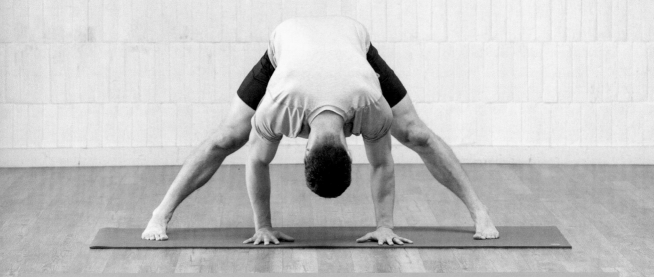

» VARIATIONS

WITH STRAP
For: added shoulder mobility

Hold the strap behind your back at shoulder width (you can bring your hands closer together as you become more flexible), and squeeze your arms as far away from your back as possible. Hug your arms toward one another to engage your scapular stabilizers (the muscles between your shoulder blades). Whether you slightly bend your elbows or lock out your arms, the important thing is to keep your shoulders in a neutral position (pulled down and back), and to avoid rounding your shoulders forward and crowding your neck.

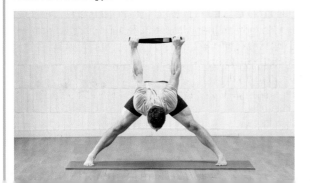

TWIST
For: thoracic mobility and rotation

Twist in one direction with your torso, and extend your arms perpendicular to the floor. Focus on twisting with your spine, and avoid bending your knees or moving your hips. If you can't get your arms straight up and down, that's okay. Keep your hips squared forward and do the best you can.

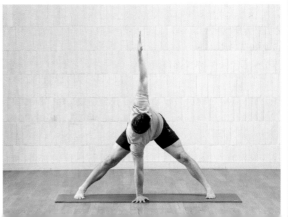

INDEX

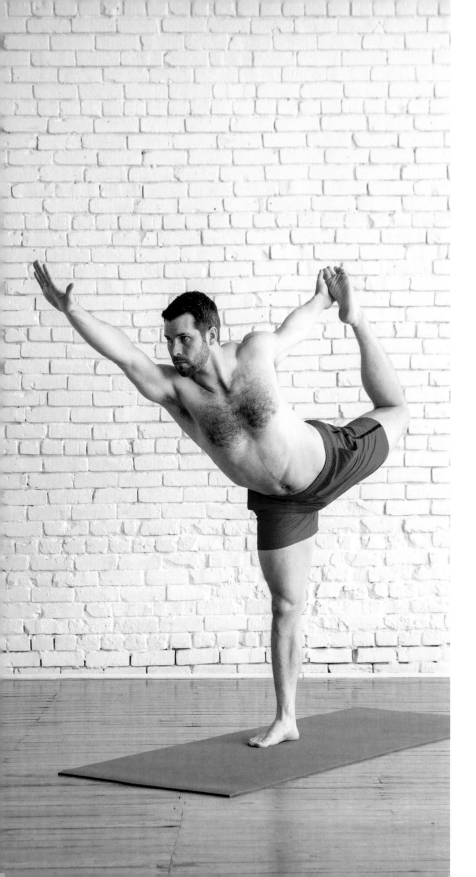

ACKNOWLEDGMENTS

I would like to first off thank DK and my editor Alexandra Andrzejewski for the opportunity to write this book. I'm a lifelong athlete, and the only reason I started yoga in the first place was because I was interested in improving my athletic performance. So for me, to be able to write the book that I would have liked to have had when I was starting out with yoga is extremely special to me.

I would also like to give a huge thank you to the superstar contributors who were involved in the making of this book. To Kelly Starrett, Brian Mackenzie, Francheska Martinez, and Nick Bare—you brought so much more to this book than I could have hoped for. Your contributions exceeded my expectations in both their thoughtfulness and quality, and your ideas nurtured my creativity to add more and more to the various sections of this book. I am so glad you were able to be part of this invaluable tool that I hope athletes will use for years and years to come.

Thank you to my parents, Brad Pohlman and Julie Callsen, for encouraging me to do my own thing, for supporting me through the ups and downs of being an entrepreneur, and for being frequent users (and reviewers) of my training programs.

Lastly, and most importantly, I would like to thank my wife, Marisa Pohlman, for her patience and understanding, allowing me to work nights and weekends for many years in order to help *Man Flow Yoga* grow from a YouTube channel into the movement and the community that it is today, for granting me time to prioritize my own fitness, and for being an inspirational mother to our son, Declan, born in June of 2020. And Declan, if you're reading this, I hope one day you'll understand that the only limits that exist are those that we allow to be placed upon ourselves, and I urge you to embrace the positive forces around you that inspire you to make your dreams come true.

PUBLISHER'S THANKS

Models: Francheska Martinez, Dean Pohlman
Digital technicians for photography: Hailey Polidori, John Davidson
Photo of Kelly Starrett on page 7: Tommy Sullivan
Photo of Brian Mackenzie on page 9: Chris Baker from WeMove Magazine
Photo of Nick Bare on page 9: Bare Performance Nutrition Team

ABOUT THE AUTHOR

Dean Pohlman has made a name for himself as the go-to internet yoga instructor for those interested in improving their fitness with yoga. Since creating the *Man Flow Yoga* YouTube channel in 2013, his videos have amassed millions of views. His internationally published book, DK's *Yoga Fitness for Men*, was published in 2018 and has been translated into French, German, and Mandarin. His DVD series, *Body By Yoga*, includes multiple top-10 best-selling programs made for all fitness levels. His website, manflowyoga.com, is one of the most popular resources on the internet for on-demand, fitness-centric yoga workouts and programs.

He has worked with physical therapists to create yoga programs for back health and spinal recovery. A former collegiate lacrosse player, his workouts and programs have been used by professional and collegiate athletes, athletic trainers, and personal trainers, and have been recommended by physical therapists, doctors, chiropractors, and other medical professionals. His work has been featured in *Muscle & Fitness Magazine, Men's Health, The Chicago Sun, New York Magazine*, and more.

Dean is an E-RYT 200 certified yoga instructor. He lives in Austin, Texas, with his wife Marisa, their son Declan, and their two dogs, Flowtron and Kaya.